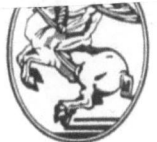

ACTA NEUROCHIRURGICA
SUPPLEMENTUM 21

Advances in Stereotactic and Functional Neurosurgery

Proceedings of the 1st Meeting
of the European Society for Stereotactic
and Functional Neurosurgery, Edinburgh 1972

Edited by
F. J. Gillingham, E. R. Hitchcock, J. W. Turner

SPRINGER-VERLAG
WIEN   NEW YORK

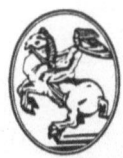

F. John Gillingham
Professor of Surgical Neurology, University of Edinburgh,
Western General Hospital and Royal Infirmary, Edinburgh

E. R. Hitchcock
Senior Lecturer in Surgical Neurology, University of Edinburgh,
Western General Hospital and Royal Infirmary, Edinburgh

J. W. Turner
Consultant Neurosurgeon, Institute of Neurological Sciences, Glasgow

With 134 Figures

Library of Congress Cataloging in Publication Data

European Society for Stereotactic and Functional
  Neurosurgery.
    Advances in stereotactic and functional neurosurgery;
proceedings of the 1st meeting of the European Society
for Stereotactic and Functional Neurosurgery, Edinburgh,
1972.

    (Acta neurochirurgica. Supplementum 21)
    Includes bibliographies.
    1. Stereoencephalotomy--Congresses. I. Gillingham,
John, 1916-   ed. II. Hitchcock, Edward Robert, ed.
III. Turner, John W., 1932-   ed. IV. Title.
V. Series. [DNLM: 1. Movement disorders--Surgery--
Congresses. 2. Pituitary gland--Surgery--Congresses.
3. Spinal cord--Surgery--Congresses. 4. Stereotaxic
techniques--Congresses. 5. Thalamus--Surgery--Con-
gresses. W1 AC8661 no. 21 / WL368 E89a 1972]
RD594.E85 1974   617'.481   74-12351

ISBN-13:978-3-211-81212-9   e-ISBN-13:978-3-7091-8355-7
DOI: 10.1007/978-3-7091-8355-7

Contents

Leksell, L., Opening Address 1

Gillingham, J., Introduction to the Scientific Sessions. Accidents in
Stereotaxy—Side-Effects or Bonus? 5

Section I

Epilepsy and Involuntary Movement Disorders

Bouchard, G., Stereotactic Operations in Generalized Forms of Epilepsy   15

Tóth, S., Zaránd, P., and Lázár, L., The Role of the Cortex and
Subcortical Ganglia in the Evoked Rhythmic Motor Activity   25

Narabayashi, H., Goto, A., Miyazaki, S., and Kosaka, K., Importance
of the Cerebellar Hemisphere in Production of Tremulous Movement or Choreo-Dystonic Movement in Monkeys   35

Andrew, J., Rice Edwards, J. M., and Rudolf, N. de M., The Placement of Stereotactic Lesions for Involuntary Movements other than
in Parkinson's Disease   39

Van Manen, J., Stereotactic Operations in Cases of Hereditary and
Intention Tremor   49

Nittner, K., and Petrovici, I. N., Contributions to the Pathogenesis of
Parinaud's Syndrome. Vertical Gaze Paralysis Following Bilateral
Stereotactic Lesion in the Interstitial Nucleus Region   57

Diemath, H. E., and Hibler, N., Vestibular Function before and after
Thalamotomy   65

Crevier, P. H., Post-Stereotactic Intracranial Haematomas   71

Section II

Hind Brain and Spinal Stereotactic Procedures

Richardson, D. E., Thalamotomy for Control of Chronic Pain   77

Laitinen, L., Arsalo, A., and Hänninen, A., Combination of Thalamotomy and Longitudinal Myelotomy in the Treatment of Multiple
Sclerosis. A Case Report   89

Mundinger, F., and Hoefer, T., Protracted Long-Term Irradiation of
Inoperable Midbrain Tumours by Stereotactic Curie-Therapy Using
Iridium-192   93

Gortvai, P., and Teruchkin, S., The Position and Extent of the
Human Dentate Nucleus   101

Tasker, R. R., Organ, L. W., and Smith, K. C., Physiological Guidelines
   for the Localization of Lesions by Percutaneous Cordotomy   111
Hitchcock, E. R., and Tsukamoto, Y., Physiological Correlates in
   Stereotactic Spinal Surgery   119
Lipton, S., Dervin, E., and Heywood, O. B., A Stereotactic Approach
   to the Anterior Percutaneous Electrical Cordotomy   125

Section III

Surgery of the Pituitary Gland and Hypothalamus

Forrest, A. P. M., Roberts, M. M., and Stewart, H. J., Pituitary Abla-
   tion by Yttrium-90   137
Angell-James, J., Hypophysectomy—The Combined Role of Neuro-
   and Rhino-Surgeons   145
Morris, L., and Wylie, I., Radiological Assessment of the Pituitary
   Gland   151
Poblete, M., and Zamboni, R., Stereotactic Pituitary Implantation
   of Radioisotopes by Transfrontal Route. 300 Cases   159
Zervas, N. T., and Hamlin, H., Stereotactic Thermal Pituitary Ablation   165
Mundinger, F., Stereotactic Curie-Therapy of Pituitary Adenomas.
   A Long-Term Follow-Up Study   169
Backlund, E.-O., Stereotactic Treatment of Craniopharyngiomas   177
Arjona, V. E., Stereotactic Hypothalamotomy in Erethic Children ...   185

Section IV

Stereotactic Techniques

Steiner, L., Leksell, L., Forster, D. M. C., Greitz, T., and Back-
   lund, E.-O., Stereotactic Radiosurgery in Intracranial Arterio-
   Venous Malformations   195
Turner, J. W., and Shaw, A., A Versatile Stereotactic System Based
   on Cylindrical Co-Ordinates and Using Absolute Measurements ...   211
Waltregny, A., Petrov, V., and Brotchi, J., Serial Stereotactic Biopsies   221
Hankinson, J., Hudgson, P., Pearce, G. W., and Morris, C. J.,
   A Simple Method for Obtaining Stereotactic Biopsies from the
   Human Basal Ganglia. A Case of Cerebral Porphyria   227
Bertrand, G., Olivier, A., and Thompson, C. J., Computer Display of
   Stereotactic Brain Maps and Probe Tracts   235
Dervin, E., Heywood, O. B., Crossley, T. R., and Dawson, B. H., The
   Use of a Small Digital Computer for Stereotactic Surgery   245
Delzanno, G. B., Redaelli, L., and Tosi, G., Mathematical Models and
   Analogic Dosimetry on Phantom in the Interstitial Radiotherapy
   of Brain Tumours with "Gamma-Med"   253
Townsend, H. R. A., Towards a Three-Dimensional Brain Model
   Stored in a Computer   265

Acta Neurochirurgica, Suppl. 21, 1—3 (1974)

Department of Neurosurgery, Karolinska Sjukhuset, Stockholm 60, Sweden

Opening Address

L. Leksell*

It is very appropriate that this first meeting of the European Society for Stereotactic and Functional Neurosurgery should be held in Edinburgh. From Sir Charles Bell up to the present time the Edinburgh school has played a prominent role among European medical centres in increasing our knowledge of the nervous system and in the progress of neurosurgery. We are grateful to our host Professor Gillingham and his colleagues, who have made important contributions to the development of stereotaxy, for taking on the task of organising this meeting and to Sir Donald Douglas and the Royal College of Surgeons for welcoming us here.

Sir Victor Horsley and R. H. Clarke laid the ground for the movement which has led to the creation of this society. After Horsleys death Clarke continued work on his stereotactic instrument and in his monograph "Investigation of the Central Nervous System" in 1920 anticipated, in his brillian introduction, virtually the whole subsequent course of stereotaxy. "The purpose of the method and instruments", writes Clarke, "is to give such practical effect as may be possible to the principle of substituting mechanical for visual direction of needles and similar fine instruments for intracranial operations, whether they are required for anatomy, physiology or surgery".

If Clarke had been able to see the program for this meeting I think he would have been very glad. The papers which we are to hear during the next two days give a clear picture of how far surgery in the depths of the brain has come as well as giving many exciting glimpses of the future. In addition to offering unlimited opportunities for exploring the functions of the human brain stereotaxy provides a practical and safe therapeutic technique which is an essential facet of neurosurgery

---

* Honorary President of the European Society for Stereotactic and Functional Neurosurgery.

and should be mastered by all brain surgeons. A priori one might expect
such intrusions into the depths of the brain to be associated with great
surgical risks. However the title of the very first paper, to be read by
Professor Gillingham, by posing the question of whether accidents in
stereotaxy might be regarded as bonuses indicates with what degree
of safety we can now probe the centre of the brain. Clarkes prophecies
of 1920 are being fulfilled. He predicted that operations for dividing
tracts in the brain would be available in the future and that in practised
hands with a 1 mm needle and 5 mm trephine scarcely would be more
serious than the extraction of a tooth.

The four sections into which the program has been divided show
how wide in the field of neurosurgery stereotaxy has already spread.
In the management of involuntary movement disorders, as also in other
branches of functional neurosurgery, the neurosurgeon must move hand
in hand with the neuropharmacologist. Progress goes in successive
waves created by the appearance of new drugs or new operating techniques. Thus pharmacology relieved a great deal of the surgeons burden
in Parkinsonism, but we shall see today how this problem has returned,
particularly in the management of tremor.

The neurosurgeons battle against intractable pain seems more promising now than hitherto. On the one hand we are on the way to a reliable
selective thalamotomy, leading to the elimination of pain without
subjecting the patient to any sensory or psychological damage. This
is a breakthrough in pain surgery that not so long ago seemed unlikely
or impossible. On the other hand the sectioning of pain tracts in the
spinal cord has been given a new revelance by the introduction of
percutaneous cordotomy. Clarke in his book already foresaw this
possibility and provides a diagram of a stereotactic instrument for
spinal surgery but it is only now that this vision has been realised.

The first stereotactic operation in man was performed at the end of
the 1920s by Kirschner who penetrated and coagulated the Gasserian
ganglion. Today the stereotactic management of tic douloureux is
becoming standard, whether by coagulation or irradiation. He also
suggested the puncturing of the hypophysis. Our program shows what
a large field this presents for exploration with limitless possibilities
both in endocrinological and in behavioural disorders.

An important recent trend has been the increasing prominence of
stereotaxy in branches of neurosurgery, which cannot be described as
functional; above all in the treatment of tumors and vascular malformations.

In the beginning there were in fact many neurosurgeons who felt
that stereotaxy was a matter for more or less esoteric neurophysiological
studies, without practical significance, but today it is evident brain

surgery in practice is composed of two main fields:—the one including the more or less classical operations under direct vision with varying degrees of optical assistance culminating in ever more intricate micro-surgery and the other the stereotactic procedures carried out blindly by mechanically controlled instruments or beams of irradiation.

Someone once said that the history of physiology is the history of the recording instruments. This applies equally to stereotaxy where advances are based on developments in instrumentation and technique. A number of new and sophisticated techniques will be presented to us tomorrow.

The first to have had the courage and foresight to use a stereotactic instrument for operations within the human brain were Spiegel and Wycis. It is largely thanks to their contribution that we gather here today. Wycis died recently, active until the last. I suggest that the society pay tribute to the memory of Henry Wycis; friend, surgeon and scientist. And that we send a telegram of appreciation and sympathy to Mrs. Wycis and also to Professor Spiegel. We turn now to the actual business and I ask the chairman of the first session, Professor Gillingham, to take over the proceedings.

Author's address: Prof. Dr. L. Leksell, Department of Neurosurgery, Karolinska Sjukhuset, Stockholm 60, Sweden.

Acta Neurochirurgica, Suppl. 21, 5—12 (1974)
© by Springer-Verlag 1974

Department of Surgical Neurology, The Royal Infirmary,
Edinburgh, Scotland

Introduction to the Scientific Sessions.
Accidents in Stereotaxy — Side-Effects or Bonus?

J. Gillingham

Stereotaxy in the human began in Edinburgh early in 1955 and I am deeply indebted to Gerard Guiot who gave my inspiration and who was my charming and persuasive mentor in those early days. The theme of my opening remarks is based on accidents in stereotaxy. Fortunately they have been uncommon but some have been curious and even beneficial. We all knew early on the problems of variation of anatomical structure within the basal ganglia and the fallability of radiological landmarks. It was the side-effects, the occasional sensory, motor or speech disturbance which forced a serious attempt to overcome the problem and led to the development of the use of physiological parameters, stimulation and depth micro-electrode recording (Gaze et al. 1964). Careful recording of side-effects and scattergrams for the plotting of lesions and these physiological techniques soon led to a better understanding of anatomical structure of cell masses and fibre interconnections.

Now stereotactic surgery has reached a high degree of precision and as we shall see, beginning to overcome the greater problem of target siting within the mobile spinal cord as well as allowing rapid extension of intracranial work into the fields of epilepsy and behaviour disorders. Although some of the newer drugs such as L-dopa have reduced the scope of the work in Parkinsonism operation still has much to offer in this disease in respect of tremor and rigidity which are often incompletely controlled by drugs. On L-dopa alone the patient has occasionally to accept limited benefit largely confined to relief of bradykinesis and this should not be as easily accepted as it now seems to be. The relative ease with which tremor is completely and lastingly abolished without side-effects by stereotaxy seems to be in danger of being forgotten. A combination of drug therapy and stereotactic surgery is still the ideal method of treatment for many patients.

However, it is the group of accidental side-effects which may pass un-
noticed and yet prove of benefit to the patient to which I want to call
attention. An unexpected part of a disease complex is relieved by a
stereotactic lesion and a new light is thrown on underlying physio-
pathological mechanisms giving an impetus to the pursuit of further
lines of research.

I would call to mind the almost immediate relief of severe and
apparently intractable pain from rigidity and the rapid disappearance
of oedema of the lower limbs due to restoration of efficiency of the
muscle/venous pump in patients with Parkinsonism during and following
operation. Less expected was the restoration of deformity which we all
had assumed to be fixed. Another unexpected bonus was the abolition
or reduction in the severity and frequency of oculo-gyric crises (Gillingham et al. 1960 and 1962). In our reported series the best results followed definitive posterior capsular lesions at 3 or 4 millimeters above
the a.c./p.c. plane, presumably because of strategic interruption of the
cortico-fugal fibres to the oculo-motor nuclei which pass there. In other
patients curious phenomena occurred. In three of our series of some
1,000 operations for Parkinsonism, oculogyric attacks appeared for the
first time immediately following succesful bilateral surgery for tremor
and rigidity. In one they were reasonably short lived. In another the
attacks were severe and frequent and in the third deviation of the
eyes upwards and to the right was almost continuous and after a
few years seem permanent. In all the attacks occurred only after the
second and contralateral lesion was made and the relief of tremor and
rigidity was strikingly complete and otherwise uncomplicated. The explanation may lie in the diversion of pathological electrical discharge
into other open pathways—in this instance a very specific one involving the oculomotor nuclei. Additional surgical lesions for the reli
ef of the complication were considered e.g. in posterior limb of the
internal capsule but precluded because of low voice volume and because improvement was anticipated.

A similar phenomenom is that of the immediate appearance of tremor
in the opposite and previously unaffected limbs when it is successfully
abolished on the first side. Also similar is the dramatic and worrying
appearance of hemiballismus following successful abolition of tremor and
rigidity. When the hemiballismus disappears—sometimes after several
weeks—the overall result for the relief of the original symptoms is
particularly good. The great paradox which exists is that hemiballismus
following an atherosclerotic vascular occlusive episode is relieved often
by a lesion in the contra-lateral ventro-lateral nucleus of the thalamus.
Yet this is an identical lesoin which when created stereotactically in
some patients with Parkinsonism results in severe hemiballismus. It does

not seem possible that our lesions—known to be discrete and made usually 3 or 4 millimetres above the inter-commisural plane—could have involved the Corpus Luysii directly but the lesion might have involved postural sensory fibres within the capsule or connections with the Corpus. Certainly since the use of depth micro-electrode recording from 1963 and greater accuracy this complication has only occurred once and on that occasion the technique of recording was known to be deficient and the lesion placed too lateral. Certainly we have never seen hemiballismuses occur following stereotactic operation for any condition other than Parkinsonism. The combination of lesions therefore, that of Parkinsonism itself and the operative one, seems important in its production. Pursuit of the problem by studing the sites of lesions of atherosclerotic hemiballismus and comparing them with those in Parkinsonism may be helpful. The problem of understanding lesions of the central nervous system may be our insistance on seeing structural alteration and our present failure to be able to record functional abnormalities of cell groups or fibres. Another problem is the difficulty of understanding and acceptance of the modification of chemical transmission by a structural stereotactic lesion.

In the early days when lesions were confined to the pallidum we sometimes observed other interesting phenomena presumably due to a temporary lesion of the lateral septal areas of the hypothalamus. For example moderately severe diabetes mellitus associated with Parkinsonism in two instances requiring heavy insulin doseage and carefully supervised diets was much better controlled after stereotactic lesions had been made and the doseage of insulin reduced to less than half of its pre-operative level. In one the benefit was short lived but in the other it was maintained for almost a year. Restoration of weight loss in Parkinsonism is a reasonably common feature following stereotactic surgery and the two phenomena may be related. Severe asthma in one instance in an elderly patient with Parkinsonism was relieved for eight months following a lesion of the globus pallidus and seborrhoeic dermatitis cleared quickly in a few patients suffering from this condition (Gillingham et al. 1960).

The association of peptic ulceration as a complication of lesions of the hypothalamus have been well documented since Cushing's Balfour lecture in 1932 on peptic ulcers and the inter-brain. 12 years ago in my own series a bank clerk of 48 years was referred by a psychiatrist for opinion regarding diagnosis and treatment of tremor of the right upper limb and neck and a severe and long-standing anxiety state. The neck tremor first appeared at the age of 22 following an emotional shock. At the age of 26 the neck tremor had improved and he joined the Army. At the age of 29 he developed a duodenal ulcer and was discharged

from the Army. When examined in 1962 we found that his neck and
limb tremor was greatly accentuated by additional anxiety. Associated
problems were an addiction to vodka and severe dyspepsia. Secretory
studies showed marked gastric hypersecretion with an overnight secretion
volume of 1.4 litres and an acid output of 100 m.Eq. Basal hourly
outputs ranged between 15 and 30 m.Eq. and post-histamine output
was as high as 110 m.Eq. Barium meal showed a large duodenal ulcer
crater. Previous treatment by sodium amytal, imipramine and antacids
failed to improve his condition and his employment was in jeopardy.
It was felt that he was under considerable emotional stress largely
because of a pre-disposed obsessional personality and that stereotactic
interruption of the thalamo-frontal projection might be the best method
of treatment for his anxiety, duodenal ulcer and also to reduce the
severity of his tremor. However, the acid response was so high that
it was regarded as a clear indication for direct surgical treatment for
the duodenal ulcer. Nevertheless it was agreed by the consultants
concerned that stereotactic interruption of the thalamo-frontal projection bilaterally in the anterior limb of the internal capsule should be
the first step. Lesions of approximately 5 mm × 5 mm × 7 mm were made
17 mm anterior to the anterior commissure, on the a.c./p.c. plane and
17 mm from the mid-line. His recovery was rapid and uneventful and
in two weeks he left hospital. His anxiety and tension were considerably
relieved. His dyspepsia rapidly disappeared and his tremor lessened
although it was not abolished. Repeated secretory studies just before
he left hospital showed little change. Three years later he reported
steady work following discharge from hospital and that he had been
promoted to a senior post as accountant with considerably more responsibility. This he managed successfully and his family life had greatly
improved. Tremor was easily controlled with a small dose of an anti-
cholinergic drug and he had few dyspeptic symptoms and no bleeding
episodes although he continued to take a small dose of antacid after
meals. His condition remained satisfactory for 12 years until a few
months ago when, at the age of 60, all his old symptoms and signs
reappeared, anxiety, tremor and dyspepsia, but much less severely
than originally. Once again barium meal confirmed the presence of an
active duodenal ulcer. Presumably it had healed in the interim period.
Secretory studies on this occasion showed a much more normal situation,
i.e. a basal secretion of 3 m.Eq. and a post-stimulatory output for
Pentagastrin of 38 m.Eq. Also the fasting serum gastrin response to
a protein meal was entirely within normal limits. The I.V. cholangio-
gram was normal.

    In retrospect the stereotactic lesions were probably too small to
have a permanent effect but on the other hand he did have twelve

very successful years in productive work and enjoyed a happy family life whereas a larger lesion might have unduly reduced his sense of responsibility. The operation was designed to reduce his anxiety and stress but in fact it also abolished the severe symptoms of a known duodenal ulcer and reduced the severity of the tremor. The decision to enlarge the lesions of the thalamo-frontal projection was held over until a trial of diazepan and antacids had been made and he has in fact made a good response.

Finally a word about intractable epilepsy. Our clinical experience of stereotactic lesions in the treatment of some 1,000 patients with Parkinsonism has been remarkable for the very low incidence of epilepsy —in fact in only 2 instances and in one of these it was strictly of the Jacksonian type and related to a scar at the site of a burr hole in the pre-motor area.

This is in accord with the observations of Williams (1965) when he postulated "that whilst focal attacks are confined to cortex and sub-cortex, focal attacks leading to a generalised convulsion abnormally activate the thalamic reticular structures which are essential to the development and diffuse spread of the general discharge. The thalamic mechanisms responsible must be intact for this process of activation and propagation of general epilepsy to occur".

Jinnai in 1963 in animal experiments endeavoured to define the conduction pathways of the epileptic convulsion "one of the most disturbing manifestations of epilepsy"—and came to the conclusion that these might be interrupted with benefit at the most strategic point, viz. the field of Forel. His subsequent clinical experience confirmed this hypothesis and a number of patients treated with stereotactic lesions in the field of Forel showed significant reduction in the frequency and severity of their attacks. We became interested in Jinnai's work because of an observation in 1958 on a patient with post-encephalitic Parkinsonism who suffered from attacks of compulsive calculation and disturbed consciousness many times a day so that he became almost inaccessible. A stereotactic operation for his Parkinsonism relieved the tremor but also reduced the frequency of his attacks to one or two a week so that he has been totally rehabilitated (Gillingham et al. 1960). The last follow-up was in 1968. The important point about this is that the area of destruction we made to relieve his tremor completely crossed the posterior limb of the internal capsule which included Jinnai's pathway but at a higher level than his point of interruption. Although two of our patients with intractable epilepsy were treated by bilateral lesions of the field of Forel mild side-effects occurred, namely temporary confusion, dysarthria and ataxia. The field of Forel and its neighbouring territory is crowded with neuronal circuits and we

Table 1. *Central Brain Lesions in Severe Epilepsy*

Patient and age	Lesion side and sites spacing in months	Follow up since last operation in months	Reduction in fit frequency and severity	Neurological state	Personality change since operations
(1) W. M. ♂ 34	(R) F. F./2M/(L) F. F.	61	by two thirds	mild ataxia (R) after second operation	none. stable invalid living at home
(2) J. D. ♂ 35	(R) V. L. Th./7M/(L)C 21M/(R) V. L. Th. 9M/(R)C	15	by half	motor paresis (L) limbs before and after operation	cerebration slowed stable living at home
(3) L. A. ♂ 30	(R) C/3M/(L)C 8M/(R) V. L. Th.	23	by half	normal before and after operation	much more stable working as gardener
(4) M. M°C ♀ 19	(L) C/6M/(R) V. L. Th.	25	by three quarters	normal before and after operations	none. stable intellectually more alert living at home
(5) A. P. ♂ 44	(R) C/3M/(L)C	29	by one quarter	mild dysarthria following second operation	more stable working in sheltered workshop
(6) D. M. ♂ 13	(R) Pal/FF/1M/Pal/FF (L)	8	by half	normal before and after operations	much less aggressive
(7) B. R. ♂	(R) Pal/FF	2	by half	right cerebrum atrophic since birth. normal before and after operations	stable normal youth
(8) D. P. ♂ 14	(R) Pal/FF	0	?	normal before and after operation	stable normal youth

turned in the next five patients to making lesions in the ansa and fasiculus lenticularis, in the capsule or adjacent ventro-lateral nucleus of the thalamus or pallidum on the basis of the observation in our patient just described with post-encephalitic Parkinsonism. Although this phenomenon of disturbance of consciousness occasionally seen in post-encephalitic Parkinsonism cannot in any way be regarded as epileptic nevertheless its relief called for further study of the possible effects of similar bilateral lesions for the relief of severe and uncontrolled epilepsy when there was no clear evidence of a constant and defined focus of discharge on electro-encephalography.

The results have shown that all patients are benefited in some degree but those helped most are those in the younger age group and who were referred earlier in their epileptic history. As well as a reduction of the frequency and severity of major fits behaviour has improved and in some minor attacks were also reduced in frequency although less markedly (Table 1).

Some of what I have touched upon will be considered in depth by those of you who are reading papers during this session. We are grateful to you for coming and promising to participate so enthusiastically. In the field of stereotactic surgery we have the great opportunity to uncover important mechanisms of disease of the central nervous system and related disorders in the process of treatment of our patients which is sometimes purposefully, and occasionally accidentally, very succesful.

Acknowledgements

It is a pleasure for me to acknowledge the assistance of Mr. J. F. Shaw for his help with the operative procedures (thalamo-frontal projection lesion) and Dr. William Sircus and Dr. J. P. A. McManus and their staff for the results of the gastro-secretory studies and their guidance in the management of the patient witn the duodenal ulcer.

References

1. Cushing, H. (1932), Peptic ulcers and the inter-brain. Surgery, Gynaecol. Obstet. *55*, 1—34.
2. Gaze, R. M., Gillingham, F. J., Kalyanaraman, S., Porter, R. W., Donaldson, A. A., Donaldson, I. M. L. (1964), Microelectrode recordings from the human thalamus. Brain *87*, 691—706.
3. Gillingham, F. J. (1962), Small localised surgical lesions of the internal capsule in the treatment of the dyskinesias. Confin. Neurol. *22*, 385—392.
4. — Kalyanaraman, S. (1965), The surgical treatment of oculogyric crises. Confin. Neurol. *19*, 237—245.
5. — Watson, W. S., Donaldson, A. A., Naughton, J. A. L. (1960), The surgical treatment of Parkinsonism. Brit. med. J. *2*, 1395—1402.

6. Gillingham, F. J., Watson, W. S. (1973), Central brain lesions in the control of intractable epilepsy. Proceedings of the Fifth European Symposium on Epilepsy. International Bureau for Epilepsy London *1973*, pp. 91—93.
7. Jinnai, D., Nishimoto, A. (1963), Stereotaxic destruction of Forel-H for treatment of epilepsy. Neurochirurgia *6*, 164—176.
8. Williams, D. (1965), The thalamus and epilepsy. Brain *88*, 539—556.

Author's address: Prof. J. Gillingham, Department of Surgical Neurology, The Royal Infirmary, Lauriston Place, Edinburgh EH 3 9 YW, Scotland.

Section I

Epilepsy and Involuntary Movement Disorders

Acta Neurochirurgica, Suppl. 21, 15—24 (1974)
© by Springer-Verlag 1974

Neurosurgical Clinic, Klinikum Steglitz,
of the Free University Berlin-West, Germany

Stereotactic Operations in Generalized Forms of Epilepsy

G. Bouchard

With 6 Figures

In recent years we have encountered a considerable number of drug resistant cases of epilepsy which does not include those of the focal or temporal lobe type we had operated on in former years. Like other neurosurgeons we also decided to treat these mainly generalized forms stereotactically. Five of the cases with an observation period of more than one year will now be described, another five with a shorter period and earlier cases unsatisfactory operated in only one hemisphere will also be considered in our final discussion.

Case 1: In spite of a daily medication of 875 mg Primidone, 180 mg Phenobarbital, 150 mg Diphenylhydantoin and 600 mg Sodiumtetraborate this 29 year old man was subjected to major and psychomotor seizures, occurring as often as ten times a week. A substitution with 800 mg Carbamacepine and 500 mg Ethosuximide proved essentially ineffective. No evidence of a genetic origin was discovered; however a severe condition of asphyxia at birth was recorded. At the age of 6 fever convulsions and at 14 generalized and temporal lobe seizures commenced, at 20 years X-radiation therapy applied to the right hemisphere on the assumption of a diffuse glioma which was never verified. EEG investigations revealed a diffuse irregularity and the production of bilateral synchronous paroxysmal slow waves during hyperventilation (Fig. 1). Improvement of only four months followed the Fornico-Amygdalotomy on the left. Additional Amygdalotomy on the right caused a reduction of attacks to short Psychomotor seizures twice a month with abortive adverse movements to the left side. Especially gratifying was the report from outside observers concerning the considerable psychological improvement in the previously existing slowness, dysphoric tension and lack of initiative.

Case 2: A 17 year old girl with two attacks a day of a prolonged dreamy state with rubbing movements of the legs was being treated with 1 g Primidone and 600 mg Carbamacepine. The attacks started in her fifth year of life. The anticonvulsive medication prevented major seizures which often led to injury. She exhibited oligophrenia with an IQ of 52 and was never able to attend school. No trace of a genetic causation could be found. Hers was a twin birth with probably extensive natal injury. The twin sister is healthy and of average intelligence. EEG findings were of diffuse irregularity rare occurrences of paroxysmal groups of slow waves during hyperventilation (Fig. 2). Subsequent to left Fornico-Amygdalotomy her attacks were reduced to between 5 and 8 attacks per month. After 9 months the frequency returned to its original level but with lasting psychological improvement as confirmed by observes. An Amygdalotomy and a VA-Thalamotomy in the right hemisphere was carried out 2 years after the first operation. Almost one and a half years later patient was free of seizures despite dose reduction of Carbamazepine. Intellectual improvement was beyond all expectation, this somewhat strong-minded egocentric patient performing all the housework for the entire family.

Case 3: A 23 year old woman suffered from a series of attacks of "absences" daily and up to three generalised tonic-clonic convulsions weekly. She received a daily dose of 1.2 g Carbamazepine, 500 mg Primidone and 1.5 g Ethosuximide or 15 mg Diazepam. Both types of attacks started in the 10th year of life since the 14th year she had increasing difficulty in school and later in work. A report of serious seizure injuries, attacks of depression, a suicide attempt, periods of paranoia and of intoxication, difficulties in speech and several dangerous status-like seizures. There was no evidence of previous brain damage but the EEG of the mother, who suffered from migraine showed pathological abnormalities. Right Fornico-Amygdalotomy produced only a small reduction of seizure frequency. Later an Amygdalotomy and VA-Thalamotomy in the left hemisphere resulted in a reduction in frequency of seizures to 1 or 2 major attaks a month always after falling asleep or before awakening. Very mild attacks of "absence" were sometimes noticed but only subjectively. Medication had to be reduced because of a paranoid state after a rather long convulsion-free period. For 9 months she remained psychologically normal and is working steadily at a finance office and according to the results of assessement after training she has good prospects of advancement (Fig. 3).

Case 4: A 25 year old woman suffered from as many as 4 major seizures a month and each day several psychomotorism or Myoclonic petit mal attacks inspite of 1.5 g Primidone and 1.5 g Ethosuximide. Medication of up to 1.2 g Carbamazepine and 2 g Ethosuximide were ineffective. Repeated severe injuries during attacks, status-like occurrences of seizures and depression were reported. Attacks of "absence" began when the patient was only 7 and major seizures began at 13. At 15 there was increasing difficulty in school and later at work. There was no evidence of acquired brain damage but a cousin of the father had epileptic fits. No improvement followed left Fornico-Amygdalotomy. Amygdalotomy and VA-Thalamotomy was performed later. Brief worsening of her general condition arose from severe menorrhagia has recurred since and at the time of upper respiratory infection there was an increase in the number of seizures. Then followed a continued improvement with now only 1 or 2 short generalized attacks with atonic falls and a few myoclonic twitching of the arms every month. The majority of the petit mal attacks disappeared and psycho-

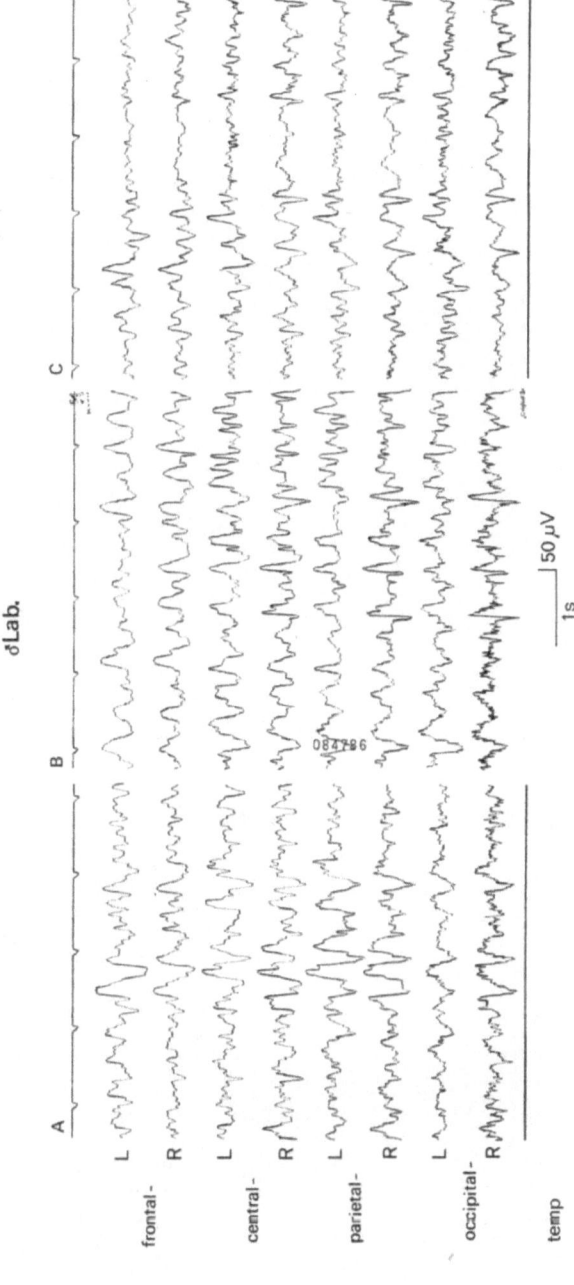

Fig. 1. EEG in Case 1. Effects of hyperventilation. A before, B after the first operation (left side), C after the second operation (right side)

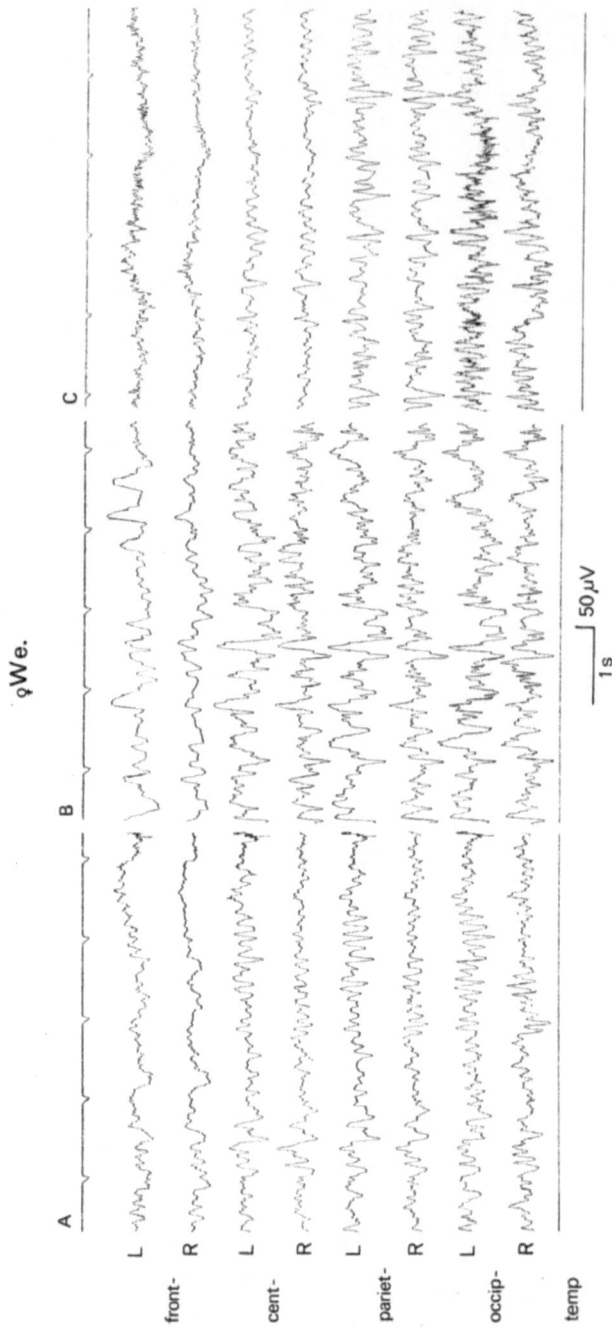

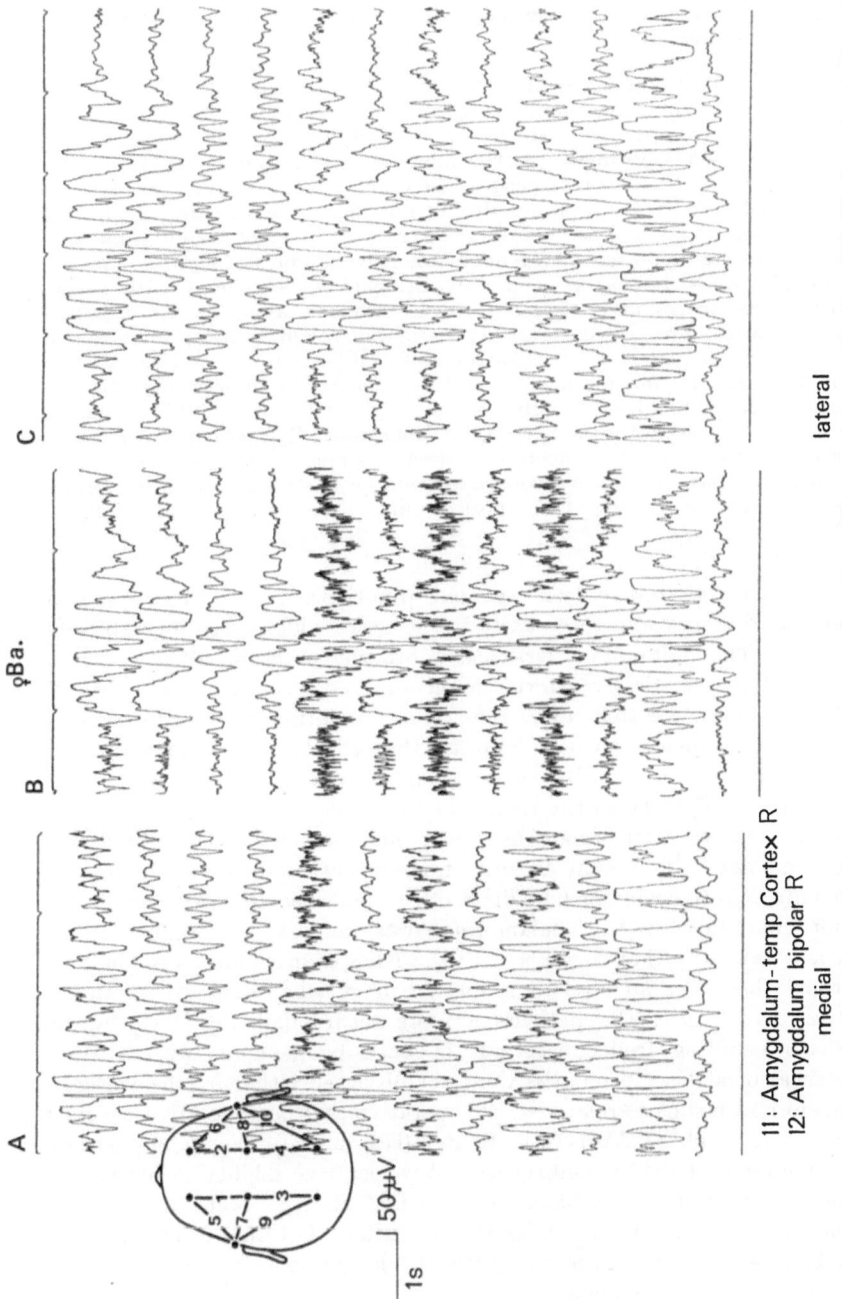

11: Amygdalum-temp Cortex R
12: Amygdalum bipolar R

medial   lateral

Fig. 3. EEG in Case 3. Spontaneous paroxysms during first operation. The average result after VA-Thalamotomy shows a disappearance of spontaneous paroxysms and a considerable reduction of those produced by hyperventilation

logical improvement with activity and self-awareness was also reported
by her husband (Fig. 4).

Case 5: A 22 year old man with 30 attacks of "absence" daily and 1 or
2 major seizures or psychomotor seizures each week mostly during sleep
and rarely during the day. He received a daily dose of 600 mg Carbamazepine and 750 mg Primidone. The addition of Ethosiuximide effected no
change. Convulsions commenced at 10 years of age. Adverse movements
to the left occurred sometimes during nocturnal convulsions. There was
no evidence of aquired cerebral damage, no possibility of finding a satisfactory explaination on assumed genetic aetiology. 2 months following Fornico-
Amygdalotomy he experienced only attacks of "absence", with severe
attacks occurring once a week, however less severe than formerly as reported
by his wife. For a year after Amygdalotomy and VA-Thalamotomy of
the left hemisphere there occurred only subjectively noticeable attacks
of "absence" lasting for only seconds at a time. A drastic reduction of
medication resulted in 3 rather severe nightly seizures within a month
which did not recur after return to the former doses. The patient was released
from his office work previous to the operations and was irregulary employed
in a warehouse. After the second operation he was reinstated in his former
position serving in a responsible post of public service with complete success
(Fig. 5).

The cases that have been excluded from this series are those operated
on more recently and those early in the series which were incompletely
treated. They fall more or less clearly into the two groups of an acquired
or a mainly genetically determined generalised form of epilepsy. All of
the patients agree that, after the second operation, the treatment was
benefical to them. To us it appears that the results obtained by the
mainly genetic forms with frequent spike wave paroxysms are not as
quite as satisfactory as the rest. The symptoms of "drop attacks" and
major seizures after falling asleep or just before awakening did not
respond and still remain an urgent therapeutic problem. Operations
in only one hemisphere had little effect, but benefits were obviously
more marked when VA-Thalamotomy was added to the original lesion.
It is noteworthy that together with the EEG changes after VA-Thalamotomy there was an obvious reduction in attacks related to emotional
stress which gave the patients a more secure daily life. Untoward
effects resulting from operations in both hemispheres with a time
interval of at least 6 months were not observed either by the patients
themselves nor close relatives. Preoperative and postoperative psychometric tests like HAWI-Test, Benton-Test and Brickenkamp-concen-
tration-endurance-test confirm this. Preoperative lability in behaviour
and tendency to depression with suicidal risks as well as paranoid
phases were not influenced by the operations but the general mental
and emotional state improves with the lessening in the number and
the severity of the attacks.

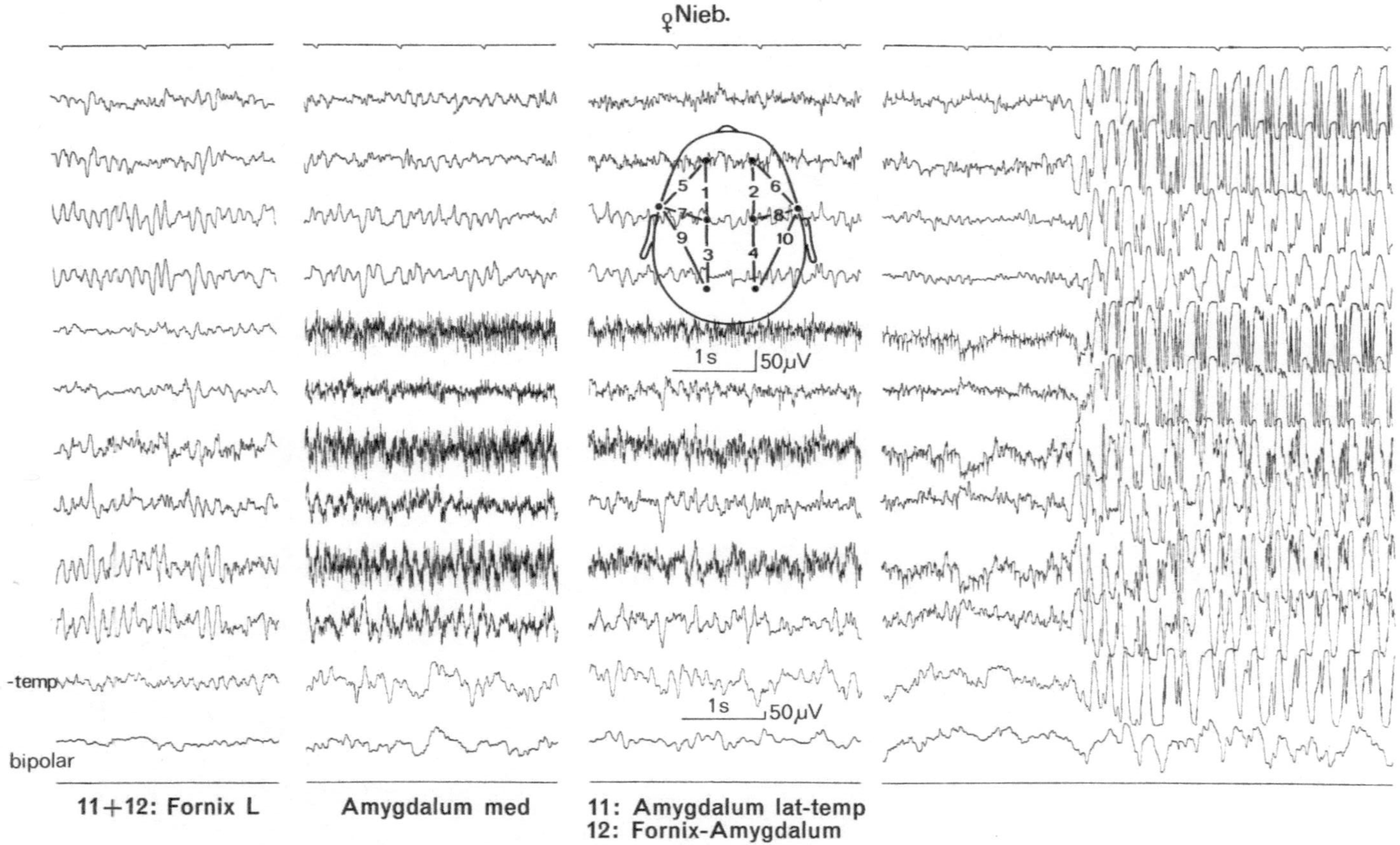
♀Nieb.
5
1
2
6
7
8
9
3
4
10
1s
50μV
-temp
bipolar
1s
50μV
11+12: Fornix L
Amygdalum med
11: Amygdalum lat-temp
12: Fornix-Amygdalum

Fig. 4. Spontaneous paroxysms in her EEG during the first operation. The average EEG findings subsequent to VA-Thalamotomy revealed a disappearance of spontaneous spike wave paroxysms and an almost complete disappearance of those resulting from hyperventilation

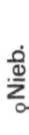

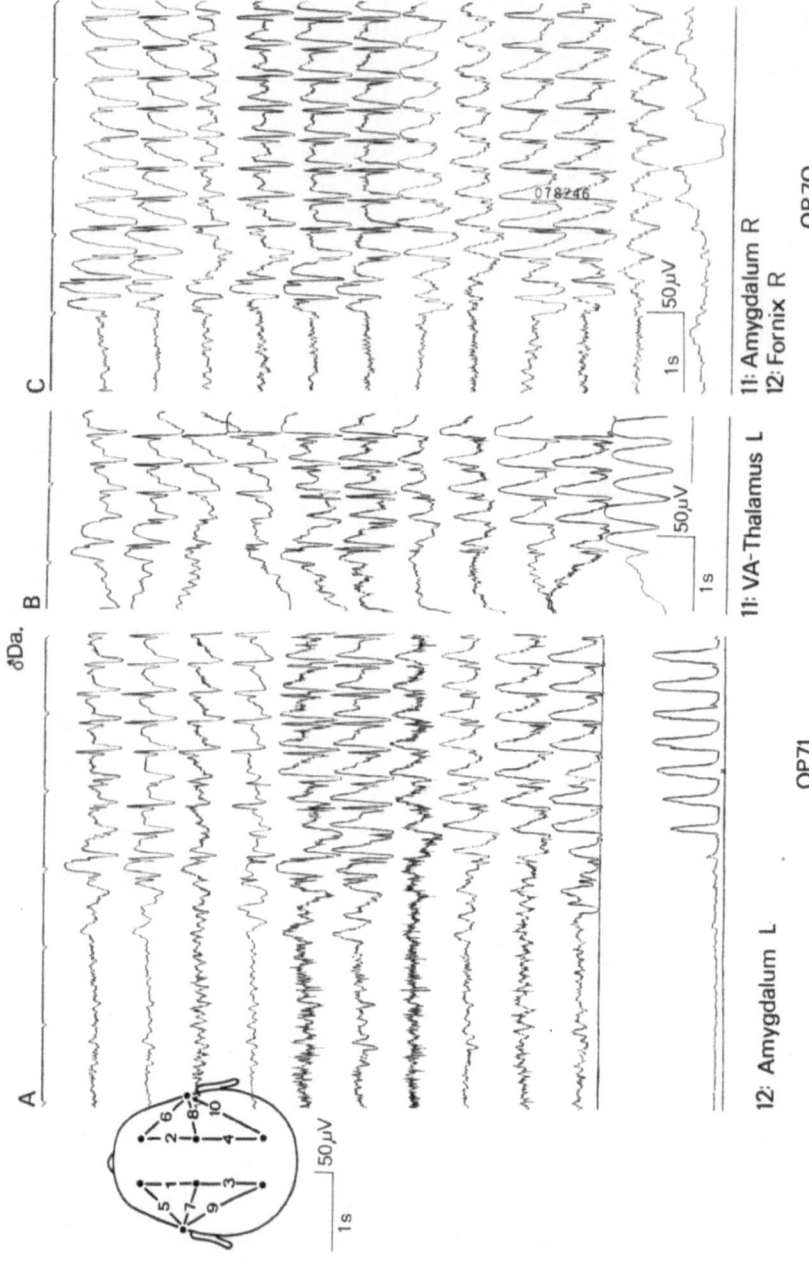

Fig. 5. Spontaneous paroxysms in his EEG during the two operations. Only once and that 3 months after the second operation spontaneous spike wave paroxysms were revealed, apart from that only occasionally during hyperventilation abortive paroxysms of second duration were registered

Stereotactic operations in cases of generalized epilepsy are reported from an experience of 20 years. We draw attention to the work of Spiegel and Wycis[9], Wada and Endo[11], Umbach and Riechert[10], Narabayashi[4], Watanabe[12], Sano[8], Jinnai and Nishimoto[2], Pardal[6], Orthner[5], Diemath and Heppner[1], Mullan[3], and Pertuiset[7].

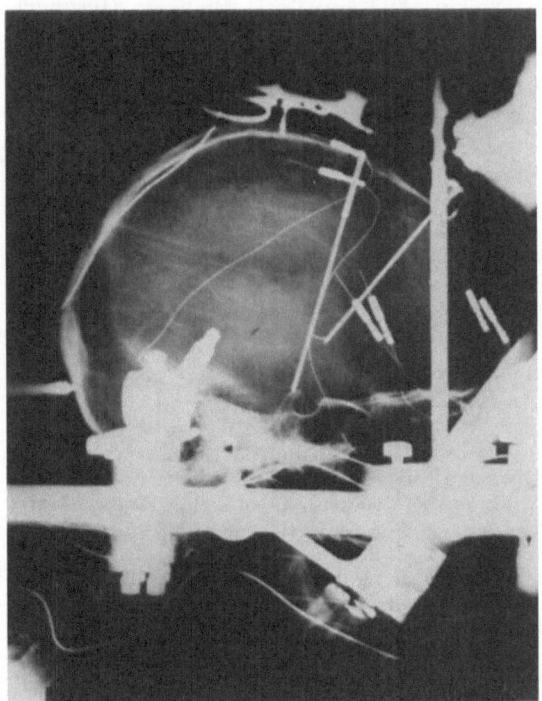

Fig. 6. The radiograph shows the intraoperative situation with inserted string electrodes for destructions in the Amygdalum, in the Fornix crossing the Commissura anterior and in the medio basal parts of VA-Thalami

The operations were performed on the Limbic System, the prefered sites being the Amygdalum, the Thalamus, on sub- and hypothalamic targets and rarely on other subcortical target points. A comparison of the different methods is not easy, because very many details with respect to the patient and the method of treatment must be considered. The results were positive and showed as in our own experience that these operative therapeutic methods should be further continued and developed.

References

1. Diemath, H. E., Heppner, F., Enge, S., Lechner, H. (1966), Die stereo-taktische vordere Cingulotomie bei therapieresistenter generalisierter Epilepsie. Confin. Neurol. *27*, 124—128.
2. Jinnai, D., Nishimoto, A. (1963), Stereotaxic destruction of Forel-H for treatment of epilepsy. Neurochir. *6*, 164—176.
3. Mullan, S., Vailati, G., Karasick, J., Mailis, M. (1967), Thalamic lesions for the control of epilepsy. Arch. Neurol. (Chic.) *16*, 277—285.
4. Narabayashi, H., Mizutani, T. (1970), Epileptic seizures and the stereo-taxic amygdalotomy. Confin. Neurol. *32*.
5. Orthner, H., Lohmann, R. (1966), Erfahrungen mit stereotaktischen Eingriffen bei Epilepsie. Dtsch. med. Wschr. *91*, 984—991.
6. Pardal, E., Morette de Pardal, M. L., Betti, O. O. (1963), Cirurgia estereotaxica de la epilepsia en los ganglios de la base. An. neurocirur-gia (B. Aires) *5*, 9.
7. Pertuiset, B., Hirsch, J. F., Sachs, M., Landau-Ferey, J., Selective stereotaxic thalamotomy in "grand mal" epilepsy. Excerpta Medica Congress series No. 193.
8. Sano, K. (1971), Effects of stimulation and destruction of the posterior hypothalamus in cases of behaviour disorders and epilepsy. In: W. Umbach: Special topics in Stereotaxis. Stuttgart: Hippokrates.
9. Spiegel, E. A., Wycis, H. T. (1962), Stereoencephalotomy Part II, S. 451—476. New York: Grune and Stratton.
10. Umbach, W., Riechert, T. (1964), Elektrophysiologische und klinische Ergebnisse stereotaktischer Eingriffe im limbischen System bei tem-poraler Epilepsie. Nervenarzt *35*, 482—488.
11. Wada, T., Endo, K. (1951), Dorsomedial thalamotomy. Preliminary report on psychic changes and therapeutic results in 35 operated cases. Folia psych. et neurol. Japonica *5*, 61.
12. Watanabe, S., Miwa, K., Takeuchi, Y. (1961), Studien über die Amygdal-otomie zur Behandlung der subcorticalen Epilepsie. Excerpta Medica Congress series *36*, 178.

Kindly assistance was given in translation from German by Dr. Bridge-water and in performing of the psychometric tests by Dr. Noell.

Author's address: Dr. G. Bouchard, Lützowstraße 20, D-1000 Berlin 30.

Acta Neurochirurgica, Suppl. 21, 25—33 (1974)
© by Springer-Verlag 1974

Institute of Neurosurgery, Budapest, Hungary

The Role of the Cortex and Subcortical Ganglia in the Evoked Rhythmic Motor Activity

S. Tóth, P. Zaránd, and L. Lázár

With 7 Figures

A number of authors (Hassler, Riechert, Mundinger, Umbach, Ganglberger 1960, Jung, Hassler 1960, Tóth 1968) have studied the problem how tremor activity was influenced by stimulation of the thalamus and pallidum. The results have shown that this stimulation may evoke, arrest or modify tremor activity. Many investigators (Guiot, Hardy, Albe-Fessard 1962, Jasper 1966, Hardy 1966) tried to find the correlation between thalamic function and tremor activity. Considering that we have found earlier that stimulation of the dentate nucleus may also evoke or modify the tremor (Tóth 1961, Tóth 1968), we suggest that the activity of a common basic structure may underlie this effect. In our opinion this basic structure is to a certain extent independent from the stimulated areas in fact it can be approached from different places with a more or less similar effect. Trying to find a possible explanation we studied this problem in patients with implanted electrodes.

In 18 patients suffering from movement disorders (Parkinsonism[6], choreo-athetosis[5], cerebellar dyskinesia[5]) or epilepsy[3] we have implanted chronic gold or platinum-irridium electrodes into the ventrolateral nucleus of the thalamus, pallidum, dentate nucleus, Brodman's area 4,6 and occasionally 8, 24 as well as into the centrum medianum. Stimulation was performed by 0.05–0.7 m/sec, 1–15 cps., 1–30 V square wave impulses. For the stimulation of the dentate nucleus we often used double stimuli of 2 m/sec interval because usually we obtained no motor responses on single stimuli. We have registered the field potentials appearing at different areas of the motor system. Parallel with it we registered the electrical activity of a muscle in voluntary contraction contralateral to the thalamic, pallidal and cortical electrodes and

ipsilateral to the cerebellar electrodes. We deemed it essential to perform the stimulation in voluntary contraction partly because with
changing the interfering activity of the functioning muscle the excitatory and inhibitory effects at the output of the motor system could
be directly registered, partly because at rest the stimuli used by us
failed to evoke motor responses appearing only during spontaneous or
voluntary activity (Tóth 1972). Besides only existing activity could

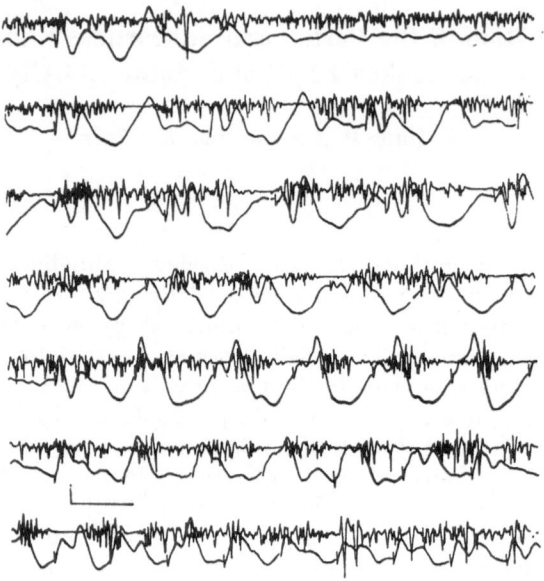

Fig. 1. E. V. 56 years old patient. Parkinsonism. The activity of the right
biceps muscle and the activities of the left 4,6 Brodmann areas during
stimulation of the left VL. Stimulation frequencies downwards: 1, 3.5,
5, 6, 7, 8 cps./30 V, 0.07 m/sec. In the electrical activity of the muscle
following the 1 cps. stimulation silent periods and rebound activity alternate
with each other after the first synchronous response. In the activity of
Brodmann 4, 6 there was a long lasting evoked potential. On raising the
frequency of stimulation the interfering electrical activity of the muscle
turns into determined groups. The frequency of these groups on 3.5, 7 cps.
stimulations follows the frequency of the stimulation and on 5, 6 cps.
stimulations the frequency is at ratio 1 : 2. On 8, 10 cps. stimulation the
muscle response becomes gradually irregular. With the changing of the
frequency of stimulation in the evoked potentials of the motor cortex there
are profound alterations with 7 cps. stimulation recruiting phenomenon
can be seen, but definitely only in the functionally active part of the evoked
potentials. Calibration for muscle activity 1.05 millivolt, for the cerebral
activity 45 microvolt. The time calibration on each recording was 100 millisec.
No tremor activity was present after the implantation of electrodes for
2–3 weeks. The investigations were carried out during this time

be transformed into grouped (tremor-like) activity. Simultaneous registration of the evoked potentials at different parts of the motor system appeared expedient because in most cases we found that they show a parallelity to peripheric muscular activity.

We have found earlier (Tóth, Zaránd, Lázár 1972) that the first wave of the evoked potential remains in most cases unchanged, while the following part—called by us the functionally active part—showed

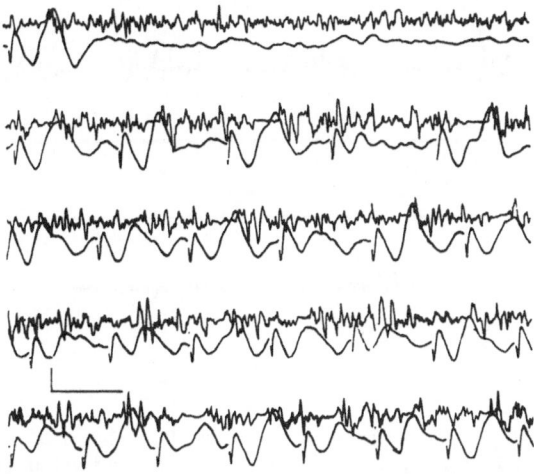

Fig. 2. The same patient as in Fig. 1. The electrical activity of the right biceps muscle and the activity of the left pallidum during the stimulation of the Brodmann 4, 6 areas on the left side. Stimulation frequencies follows each other 1, 6, 7, 8, 9 cps. (15 V, 0.05 m/sec) downwards. The continous activity of the right biceps muscle mainly during the 6, 8 cps. stimulations transforms into grouped activity. The frequency of the tremor-like muscle activity compared to the frequency of the stimuli, with the stimulations of 6, 8 cps. is at a ratio 1 : 2 and in the stimulation of 9 cps. 1 : 1. With the gradual increasing frequency of stimulations the functionally active part of the evoked-potentials are gradually changing. Calibration for muscle activity (750 microvolt), for the cerebral activity (15 microvolt)

significant changes depending on the grade of innervation or the type of stimulation.

No tremor activity was present in our patients with Parkinsonism because the implantation of electrodes for long term studies was always followed by complete cessation of tremor activity for 2–3 weeks.

We have found that in our patients with stimulation of these parts of the motor system the interfering electrical activity of each muscle (contralateral to the thalamic, pallidal and cortical electrodes and ipsilateral to the cerebellar electrodes) can be transformed into grouped (tremor-like) activity. As a rule in this state neither the electrical activity of the muscle nor the clinical picture can be distinguished from parkinsonian or cerebellar tremor. This phenomenon could equally be obtained in patients suffering from Parkinsonism or other movement disorders as well as in epileptic patients with a probably intact motor system.

Tremor-like activity could be most readily evoked by the stimulation of the ventrolateral nucleus of the thalamus (Figs. 1, 2, and 3) rarely by

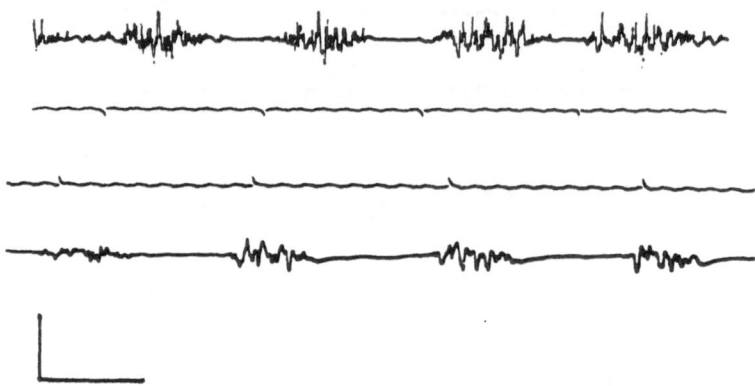

Fig. 3. V. J. 16 years old patient. Epilepsy. The electrical activity of the left biceps muscle developes into clear tremor-like activity during the stimulation of the thalamus (VL). It is seen in the upper part of the recording. The same picture can be seen during the stimulation of area 24 of Brodmann in the lower part of the picture. The sites of the stimulation are marked on the parallel line. Parameters of the thalamic stimulation (0.7 m/sec, 20 V, 7 cps.). Parameters for the stimulation studies of area 24 of Brodmann (0.7 m/sec, 25 V, 6 cps.). Calibration for the muscle during thalamic stimulation (0.75 millivolt for area 24 stimulation) (450 microvolt)

stimulation of the dentate nucleus (Figs. 4, 5). It has often occurred on the stimulation of the pallidum but rarely on the stimulation of other structures that the large synchronous action potentials of the muscles following stimuli did not disappear on raising the frequency of the stimulation and thus the tremor-like picture failed to develop in the electric response and clinically serial twiching could be observed (Fig. 6).

On stimulation of the ventrolateral nucleus, of the pallidum and of the cortical areas grouped tremor-like activity most often appeared at the 3–7 cps. frequency band. Tremor-like activity either corresponds to the frequency of stimulation or lags behind in at a ratio 2 : 1 (Figs. 1, 2, and 3). With stimulation of the dentate nucleus tremor-like activity most frequently appeared at a frequency band of 5–10 cps. It either followed the frequency of stimulation or was faster with a ratio of 2 : 1 (Figs. 4 and 5). Changes of the frequency of the stimulation were accompanied by profound changes in the functionally active part of the

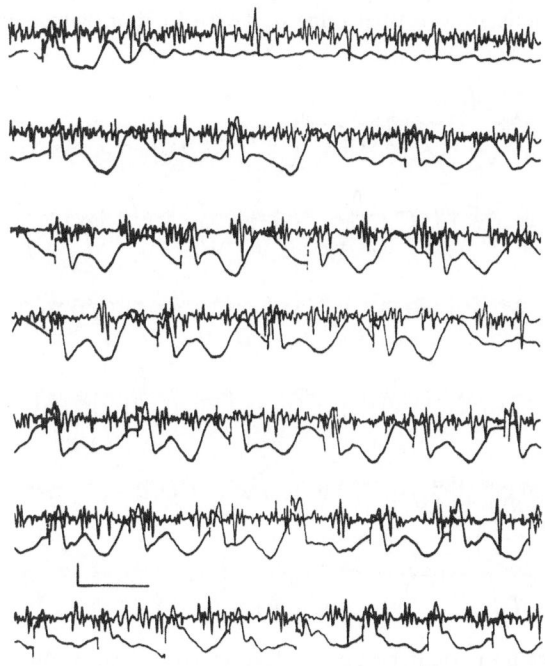

Fig. 4. The same patient as in Fig. 1. The activity of the right biceps muscle and the activity of the left VL nucleus of the thalamus during stimulation of the right dentate nucleus. The frequencies of stimulation from top to the bottom 1, are 3.5, 5, 6, 7, 8, 10 cps. (0.05 millisec., 30 V). The pronounced evoked-potential on 1 cps. stimulation can be clearly seen. No definite change in the muscle activity occurs. By raising the frequency of stimulation the electrical activity of the muscle gradually become grouped. The grouping becomes regular on 8, 10 cps. stimulation. The grouped activity and the frequency of stimulation are at a ratio 2 : 1. The functionally active part of the evoked-potentials gradually changes on raising the stimulation frequency. Calibration for muscle activity (1.05 millivolt) for cerebral activity (15 microvolt)

field potentials (Figs. 1, 2, 4, and 5). We shall report on them at a later date.

In the case of existing spontaneous tremor, tremor activity could be most readily elicited in the resting state with stimulation at its own frequency.

Single stimulation of the chosen parts of the motor system were followed by signs of excitation and inhibition in muscular electrical activity. The excitatory and inhibitory periods most often appeared in the form of synchronous waves or groups of potentials with higher amplitudes followed by silent periods and rebound activity. The silent-rebound periods may return once or twice in damped form. The time

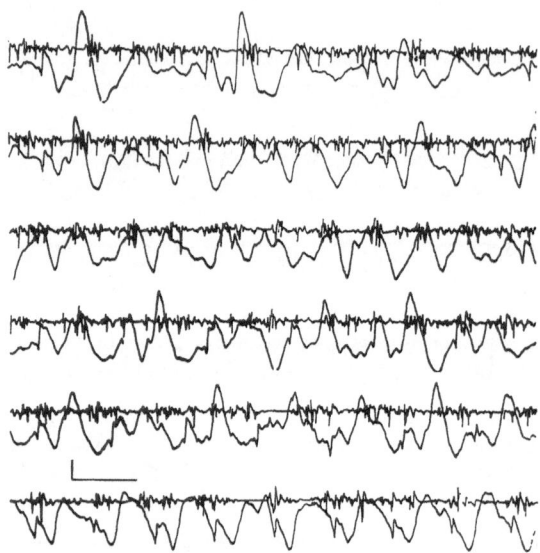

Fig. 5. The same patient as in Fig. 1. Activity of the right biceps muscle and the activity of the Brodmann 4, 6 areas during stimulation of the right dentate nucleus. Downwards 3.5, 5, 6, 7, 8, 10 cps. stimulation frequencies (0.05 m/sec, 30 V), with a double stimulus of 2 millisec interval. The motor responses are seen earlier than on the Fig. 4, but in fact they are the same. The change of the functionally active part of the evoked-potentials are clearly shown on raising the frequency of stimulation. Calibration for muscle activity (1.05 millivolt) for cerebral activity (15 microvolt)

and intensity of these periods may change within certain limits depending on the grade of innervation and on the parameters of stimulation. The constant part of responses is within 60–120 m/sec, 1 cps. stimulation (Figs. 1, 2, and 6), 3.5 cps. stimulation (Fig. 5). The changes most probably correspond to the alterations in the polysynaptic spinal reflex arc under the control of the stimulated centres. The uniformity of the responses obtained by stimulation of the different areas implies a type of convergence and to some extent similar responses can be obtained by peripheric stimulation Hoffmann (1922), Granit (1950), Granit, Kellerth, Sumski (1966), Faganel (1971), Hugon, Bonnet, Roll (1971).

Generally the grouped, tremor-like activity developes from the peripheral motor response so that the synchronous electric response decreases, than disappears on raising the frequency of stimulation and the subsequent rebounds—preceeded and followed by silent periods—in-

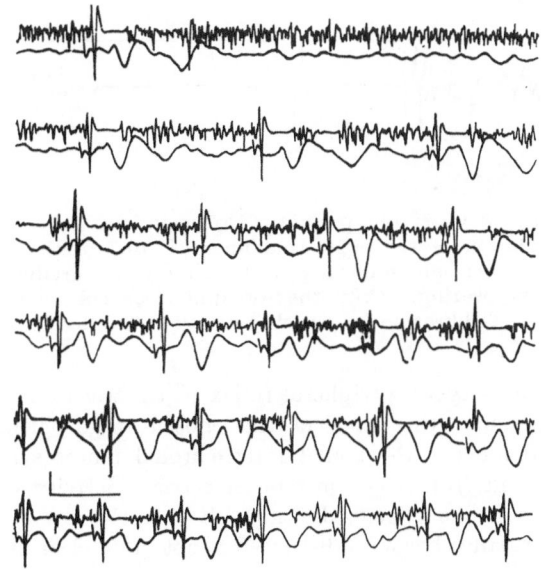

Fig. 6. The same patient as in Fig. 1. Electrical activity of the right biceps muscle and activity of the left 4, 6 Brodmann areas during stimulation of the left pallidum. Frequency of stimulations downwards 1, 3.5, 5, 6, 7, 8 cps. (0.05 millisec, 15 V). At all frequencies following stimuli the large synchronous action potentials of the muscle are pronounced therefore tremor-like activity cannot develop. Calibration for muscle activity (1.05 millivolt) for cerebral activity (45 microvolt)

creases (Fig. 7). This state is maintained by the subsequent stimulations. The development of the rhythmic responses not synchronous with the frequency of stimulation showed a somewhat different pattern.

We do not intend to reduce the mechanism of parkinsonian tremor and of tremors of other origin to a common denominator with the above. However it seems fairly probable, that the conditions of the oscillation time of the excitation and inhibition periods in the spinal reflex arc fundamentally determine the mechanism of tremor. The same time patterns determine the resonance frequency band of the tremor-like activity following stimulation of different parts of the motor system.

Often the stimuli falling in the middle of the silent period maintained the tremor-like activity best (Fig. 1 7 cps. stimulation; Fig. 3 VL stimulation). This appears to support a control through the gamma neurons (Stern, Ward Jr. 1960, Ohye, Kubota, Hongo, Narabayashi 1964, Laitinen, Ohno 1970) more probably through the spinal interneurons. The latter is supported by the fact that we never could elicit

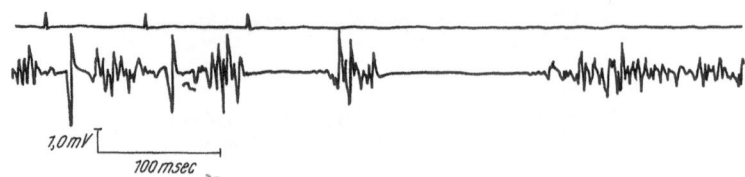

Fig. 7. Sz. B. 28 years old patient. Epilepsy. In the left biceps muscle during stimulation of the right thalamus VL (0.7 millisec, 20 V, 11 cps.) synchronous potentials following each stimuli are gradually decreasing and than disappearing. Only the rebound electrical activity is present. Calibration for muscle activity (1.0 millivolt)

tremor-like activity by peripheral reflex or electrical stimuli. Through stimulation, under the drive of the chosen target primarily of the ventrolateral nucleus the spinal interneuronal motor system becomes unbalanced and from the continous electrical activity of the muscle grouped, tremor-like activity develops. How in the case of parkinsonian tremor this balance becomes disturbed is not quite clear as yet.

References

1. Faganel, J. (1971), Electromyographic analysis of human flexion reflex components. 4e Congres International d'Electromyographie Bruxelles 1971. Résumé de communication et des rapports, 47—48.
2. Granit, R. (1950), Antigenic inhibition. J. EEG clin. Neurophysiol. *2*, 417—424.
3. — Kellerth, J. O., Sumski, A. J. (1966), Intracellular antigenic effects of muscular contraction on extensor motoneurons. The silent period. J. Physiol. (London) *182*, 484—503.
4. Guiot, G., Hardy, J., Albe-Fessard, D. (1962), Délimination précise des structures sous-corticales et identification de noyaux thalamiques chez l'homme par l'electrophysiologie Stereotactique. Neurochirurgie *5*, 1—18.
5. Hardy, J. (1966), Electrophysiological localisation and identification. 2nd Symposium on Parkinson's Disease, Washington, 1964. J. Neurosurg. *24*, Suppl. Part. II, 410—414.
6. Hassler, R., Riechert, T., Mundinger, F., Umbach, W., Ganglberger, J. A. (1960), Physiological observations in stereotaxic operations in extrapyramidal motor disturbances. Brain *83*, 337—350.

7. Hoffmann, P. (1922), Untersuchungen über die Eigenreflexe (Sehnenreflexe) menschlicher Muskeln. Berlin: Springer.
8. Hugon, M., Bonnet, M., Roll, P. (1971), Réflèxes Proprioceptifs et Exteroceptivs chez l'Homme Normal. 4e Congres International D'Electromyographie Bruxelles, 1971. Resumé de communications et des rapports.
9. Jasper, H. H. (1966), Recording from microelectrodes in stereotactic surgery from Parkinson's Disease. 2nd Symposium on Parkinson's Disease, Washington. 1964. J. Neurosurg. 24, Suppl. Part. II, 219—221.
10. Jung, R., Hassler, R. (1960), The extrapyramidal motor system. In: Handbook of Physiology. Sect. I: Neurophysiology. Ed. by Field, J., Magoun, H. W., Hall, V. E., American Physiological Society, Washington, 1960, Vol. II, 863—927.
11. Laitinen, L. V., Ohno, Y. (1970), Effects of thalamic stimulation and thalamotomy on the H-reflex. J. EEG and clin. Neurophysiol. 28, 586—591.
12. Ohye, C., Kubota, K., Hongo, T., Narabayashi, H. (1964), Ventrolateral subventrolateral thalamic stimulation. Arch. Neurol. 11, 427—434.
13. Stern, J., Ward, A. A., Jr. (1960), Inhibition of the muscle spindle discharge by ventrolateral thalamic stimulation. Arch. Neurol. 3, 193—204.
14. Tóth, S. (1961), Effect of removal of the dentate nucleus on the parkinsonien syndrome. J. Neurol. Neurosurg. Psychiat. 24, 143—147.
15. — (1968), Az extrapyramidalis mozgászavarok mütéti kezelése. (Thesis), p. 114. Budapest: Akadémiai könyvtár.
16. — (1970), Proceedings, International Symposium on Neurophysiology in Man, Paris, 1971. Excerpta Medica, in Press.
17. — Zaránd, P., Lázár, L. (1972), Study of cortical and subcortical connections within the motor system in man. 27th Congress of the Hungarian Society for Neurology and Psychiatry, p. 200. Budapest: Publishing House of Hungarian Academy.

Author's address: Dr. S. Tóth, Amerikai u. 57, Budapest XIV, Hungary.

Acta Neurochirurgica, Suppl. 21, 35—38 (1974)
© by Springer-Verlag 1974

Department of Neurology, Juntendo Medical School, Bunkyo-Ku, Tokyo,
Japan

Importance of the Cerebellar Hemisphere in Production of Tremulous Movement or Choreo-Dystonic Movement in Monkeys

H. Narabayashi, A. Goto, S. Miyazaki, and K. Kosaka

Experience of the use of stereotaxic surgery in Parkinsonism and for different kinds of tremulous movements, and analysis of the results have led to the conclusion that the surgical target for tremor and that for rigidity is slightly different in respect of localization within the thalamus. Tremor is located posteriorly in the Ventralis Intermedius Nucleus (Vim) and rigidity is anteriorly in the Ventralis Lateralis Nucleus (VL). In our several previous reports, differentiation of these two subnuclei was discussed in detail.

As described by Nauta and Mehler in monkeys, by Do.mont et al. (1968) in cats and by Hassler (1949) in human studies, the pallidum and cerebellar structures send their projections to the thalamus in slightly different areas. Kusama (1910) suggested that pallidal efferents project to the VL and VA (ventralis anterior nucleus) and the more posterior area from VL, presumably the Vim area, receives more of the cerebellar afferent inflow. Clinical and functional correlation or interrelation between these two systems is specially interesting and the following experiments in monkeys were tried.

Stimulation of VL was carried out in six macaque monkeys (Table 1). Using the stereotactic technique for placement of the electrode of an atlas of the monkeys brain. Accurate siting was confirmed by VL-evoked cortical responses on the EEG. One monkey was sacrificed for postmortem study afterwards.

In four, the cerebellar hemispheres including the dentate nucleus were completely removed by suction, bilaterally in three and unilaterally in one. For the transient period of two to four weeks after operation, the animal presented the typical hypotonia of its extremities and

3*

dysmetria, which then gradually subsided to almost subnormal motor activities. All were kept and fed for more than several months (usually more than four) after the procedure and were then subjected to stimulation of VL. Tremor was reproduced by high frequency stimulation (60 c/s, 0.5 m/sec, 12–14 V) of VL in all four monkeys with cerebellar surgery and never in two normal monkeys used as controls. Tremor produced was of rhythmic, regular shaking of the arm and leg and contraction of facial muscles with a frequency of 4 to 6 per seconds and was always produced contralateral to the VL nucleus stimulated.

Table 1. *Series of Experiments on Tremor Production in 6 Monkeys*

VL Stimulation		Tremor
Monkey 15	bilaterally cerebellar hemispherectomized	+ +
Monkey 22	bilaterally cerebellar hemispherectomized	+ +
Monkey 24	bilaterally cerebellar hemispherectomized	+
Monkey 26	right cerebellar hemispherectomized	+

In two control monkeys (non-operated on cerebellum), tremor never appeared.

Monkey 30, 31		—

These findings would suggest that some secondary functional changes in the posterior VL area in the chronic stage after cerebellar hemispherectomy would be necessary for the manifestation of tremor in addition to VL stimulation.

The normal monkeys used as controls did show some stiffness on the contralateral extremities to stimulation during the period of high frequency stimulation of VL but never tremulous movement. Harmaline, which is known to induce rigidity pharmacologically causes a shivering-like slight tremor even in normal monkeys but the more vigorous rhythmic movement resembling marked tremor is seen more commonly when it is applied to monkeys subjected to cerebellar hemispherectomy after some months. Poirier suggested that the lesion within a rubro-olivo-cerebello-rubral loop would be a necessary condition in order to produce tremor in monkeys.

From these experiments in animals, the two motor symptoms of Parkinsonism, rigidity and tremor, should be considered quite independently yet the correlation between the two symptoms should also be important.

The second topic is the pharmacologically induced choreo-dystonia in monkeys. In the course of L-Dopa treatment for Parkinsonism, the choreo-dystonic type of hyperkinesis is the well known complication. It is also established that the choreic movement of Huntington's chorea can definitely be worsened by a low-dosage of L-Dopa and this is now applied for detection of latent or early cases of Huntington's disease. The following experiment was designed to produce a similar type of hyperkinesis in monkeys.

The combination of L-Dopa (100–200 mg intravenously) and the

Table 2. *Series of Experiments on Pharmacologically Induced Choreo-Dystonic in 6 Monkeys*

(RO 4–4602 10–20 mg i.p., l–Dopa 100–200 mg i.v.)

1. Control

Monkey 27	+
Monkey 30	+ +
Monkey 31	+ +

2. Bilaterally cerebellar hemispherectomized

Monkey 22	—
Monkey 28	—

3. Right cerebellar hemispherectomized

Monkey 29	choreodystonia + mainly on the left side of the body

peripheral inhibitor of dopa-decarbosylase R 04–4602 (10–20 mg intraperitoneally), was used in 6 monkeys (Table 2). On average monkeys used weighed between 5 to 7.5 kg in body weight.

Typical choreo-dystonic movement started to appear about in 15 to 20 minutes and continued for about one to two hours. The abnormal movement was observed mainly in the neck and shoulder area and in some in the peroral area. Extremities were much less affected. Quick or tonic contraction of the head posteriorly associated with torsion of shoulder was most common. Sustained opening of mouth or rhythmic biting movements became difficult. On a few occasions the fingers showed an extensor twitch and the feet showed twitching inversion movements at the ankle.

The two normal control monkeys showed this phenomena quite regularly using the dosage previously described but the three monkeys with bilateral cerebellar hemispherectomy did not. However the one monkey after unilateral hemispherectomy presented symptoms more on the contralateral side of the body. This would suggest the possibility of aleviation or lessening choreo-dystonic movements by dentatotomy.

These two experiments in monkeys suggest the possible rôle of the cerebellar hemispheres in certain types of hyperkinesis.

References

Dormont, J. F., Ohye, C., Albe-Fessard, D. (1968), Comparison of the relationships of the nucleus entopeduncularis and brachium conjuncti-vum with the thalamic nucleus ventralis lateralis of the cat. Third Symposium on Parkinson's Disease, pp. 103—111.

Hassler, R. (1949), II. Mitteilung. Weitere Bahnen aus Pallidum, Ruber, vestibulärem System zum Thalamus; Übersicht und Besprechung der Ergebnisse. Arch. Psychiat. *182*, 786—818.

Klawans, H. L., Barbeau, A., Paulson, G. W. (1972), Use of L-Dopa in early detection of Huntington's chorea. Centennial Symposium on Huntington's chorea, Columbus, Ohio, March 1972.

Kusama, T. (1970), Fiber connections of the extrapyramidal system. Progress of Medicine, (in Japanese) *75*, 71—78, 183—190, 378—385.

Larochelle, L., Bedard, P., Boucher, R., Poirier, L. (1970), The rubro-olivo-cerebello-rubral loop and postural tremor in the monkey. J. Neurol. Sci. *11*, 53—64.

Mones, R. J. (1972), The experimental production of chorea in monkeys. Centennial Symposium on Huntington's Chorea, Columbus, Ohio, March 1972.

Narabayashi, H. (1968), Muscle tone conducting system and tremor con-cerned structures. Third Symposium on Parkinson's Disease, Edin-burgh, 246—251.

— (1968), Functional differentiation in and around the ventrolateral nucleus of the thalamus based on experience in human stereoencephal-otomy. J. Hopkins Med. J. *122*, 295—300.

— (1968), Analysis of tremor in human cases and experimental tremor in monkeys. Advances in Neurological Sciences, in press (in Japanese).

Ohye, C., Kubota, K., Hongo, T., Nagao, T., Narabayashi, H. (1964), Ventro-lateral and subventrolateral thalamic stimulation. Arch. Neurol. *11*, 427—434.

Sax, D. S., Butters, N., Tomlinson, E. B., Feldman, R. G. (1972), Caudate nucleus lesions and L-Dopa, a model for Huntington's chorea. Centennial Symposium on Huntington's Chorea, Columbus, Ohio, March 1972.

Authors' address: H. Narabayashi, M.D., A. Goto, M.D., S. Miyazaki, M.D., K. Kosaka, M.D., Department of Neurology, Juntendo Medical School, Bunkyo-ku, Tokyo, Japan.

Acta Neurochirurgica, Suppl. 21, 39—47 (1974)

The Middlesex and Charing Cross Hospitals, London, and
Oldchurch Hospital, Romford, Essex, England

The Placement of Stereotaxic Lesions
for Involuntary Movements other than
in Parkinson's Disease

J. Andrew, J. M. Rice Edwards, and N. de M. Rudolf

Introduction

This report concerns 37 thalamotomies in 25 patients. Table 1 shows
the various diagnoses.

Table 1. *Classification of Patients*

Essential Tremor	
Simple	3
Associated with spasmodic torticollis	2
Intention Tremor	
Aetiology uncertain	3
Due to disseminated sclerosis	4
Spasmodic torticollis or retrocollis	6
Torsion Dystonia	
Unilateral	3
Generalised and associated with spasmodic	
torticollis	1
Hemiballismus	1
Huntington's Chorea	2
Total	25

A word is needed about the classification of tremors which is clouded
at the present time. Some neurologists distinguish between postural
and intention tremor; others consider this too neat, because the two
may occur together. Some would even regard postural tremor as a type
of intention tremor affecting axial muscles. Essential tremor is usually
regarded as a postural tremor (Marshall 1968), sometimes as an intention

tremor (Cooper 1969). In truth, movement of the arm in this condition may or may not involve an increase in the tremor of its distal part as it nears its target. As essential tremor is a clear clinical entity we have isolated it.

The second group comprises severe intention tremors. In fact, all the patients in the first sub-group and two of those with disseminated sclerosis also had marked postural tremor. Furthermore, two in the first sub-group had tremor at rest as well. Thus some had mixed tremors, but as severe intention tremor was the dominant aspect, they are so classified. These mixed tremors have been called superior cerebellar peduncle or red nucleus types, but these terms are best avoided as their pathological basis is insecure and their definition imprecise.

Method

In our technique, the Watkins perforated sphere was fixed between plates near the coronal suture approximately 4 cm from the midline using the Rivers-Bennett stereotaxic frame. The 13 perforations in the sphere were 3 mm apart in approximate sagittal and coronal planes. The reference planes, defined by contrast films, were the vertical transverse plane through the posterior border of the interventricular foramen of Monro, the horizontal plane between the foramen and the posterior commissure, and the midline. A check probe was passed to a calculated depth down the central hole, and, after further X-rays, any necessary change was in the calculation. One or more targets were selected according to the diagnosis, as described later.

Because of the variability of the borders of thalamic nuclei in relation to the reference planes, the targets calculated from the variability atlas of Andrew and Watkins (1969) were if possible confirmed physiologically.

Single unit recording was carried out using a bipolar micro-electrode with a tip of less than 30 micra, which records waves as well as unit spike discharges. A micrometer, fixed to the sphere, propelled the electrode; insertion was usually halted at each millimetre, the activity observed in more detail and tests for evoked responses applied.

Alternative or supplementary testing was by electrical stimulation with a unipolar electrode having a tip 1 mm long and 1 mm in diameter, and a 50 c/sec sine wave variable in $\frac{1}{4}$ volt steps. Both recording and stimulation might be carried out along more than one parallel trajectory. The results might indicate a site for a lesion where a particular response had been found, or serve to determine a lesion site elsewhere.

Our lesion is smaller than that made by some authors but can be equally effective. It is produced with an electrode tip of 5 or 6 mm and 1 mm diameter, and a radiofrequency current which raises the temperature at the tip to 66 °C for 150 seconds. The resulting lesion is 6 or 7 mm in length and forms an oblate spheroid with maximum diameter of 3–4 mm.

Results

To compare the success of the various methods for determining lesion placement, all thalamotomies in which the outcome of the operation on the right and left sides can be assessed are summarized, irrespective of diagnosis, in Table 2. Cases excluded are midline or generalized conditions in which the separate effects of right and left lesions, localized by differing methods, cannot be assessed because the second side had to be treated before the result on both sides was complete. "Good", "fair" and "poor" are defined by degree of improvement and incidence of side-effects, if any. For example, "good" means complete relief with only mild side-effects or none, or at least moderate relief without side-effects. It is seen that there is no obvious difference between the

Table 2. *Cases in which Methods of Localization of Lesions can be Assessed in Terms of Results*

Thalami with lesions localized by: —	Total	Results		
		Good	Fair	Poor
Recording	6	4	2	0
Stimulation	11	10	0	1
Recording and Stimulation	8	4	1	3
Anatomical Coordinates alone	5	4	0	1

methods of localization, and that, even by the atlas alone, the success rate is reasonably high, though numbers are small. It does not appear that recording is greatly superior to stimulation, despite the presumed inaccuracy of the latter owing to unpredictable stimulus spread. However, it is possible that the newer technique is not yet being used to full advantage. In this series, evoked responses have been taken as guides in 18 thalamotomies, while in three the amplitude of spontaneous activity was employed, and in two tremor bursts. These spontaneous bursts of firing in the tremor-frequency band occurred in only three of these 12 patients with tremor, but in 40% of 55 tremor cases studied previously, of whom only eight were non-Parkinsonian (Andrew and Rudolf 1972). The final site for one or more lesions was based on the recording results in relation to our concept of physiological representation in the thalamus, derived from a larger series including many Parkinsonian patients, which we have reported (Rudolf 1969, Andrew and Rudolf 1972, 1973). Refinement of these somatotopic data and perhaps more use of additional recording variables, such as "slow" waves, may enhance the value of recording. Certainly the present

analysis has revealed that negative findings are usually explicable by
the variability study—the electrode tip was simply not within the
average boundaries of the appropriate nucleus.

In all cases of tremor, as well as in Huntington's chorea, hemiballismus and unilateral torsion dystonia, our policy was to make a lesion
in the anterior part of the ventralis caudalis externus (V.c.e.), that is,
in the region of evoked responses, or where sensory effects were obtained
by an electrical stimulus, or where the atlas showed the average V.c.e.
to lie. If necessary, a second lesion was made, usually more anterior
in ventro-intermedius (V.im.) and 13 mm from the midline for the arm,
or 15–16 mm for the leg. It is emphasized that from the atlas and
variability study one can derive only the nucleus or nuclei, in which a
lesion, centered at given co-ordinates, is most likely to lie. In the case,
for example, of the ventro-caudalis internus (V.c.i.) or centro-medianum
(Ce.M.) this assessment can be reached directly, because boundaries
with standard deviations are given; on the other hand average boundaries for the V.c.e. and V.im. are not available although their general
position is indicated. However, since their relationships to the Ce.M.,
V.c.i. and lateral thalamic mass are well known from various published
atlases, we have judged their positions on this basis.

The alternative method of quoting co-ordinates was considered but
rejected owing the the differing reference points, scaling factors and
co-ordinate systems employed in stereotaxic surgery. However, the
mean positions, with standard deviations, of the centres of the most
numerous single-nucleus lesions were as follows (the tables represent in
millimetres the distances behind the interventricular foramen, above
the horizontal reference plane and lateral to the midline respectively):

$$V.im.: \quad 12.4 \pm 1.1, \; 2.3 \pm 0.8, \; 13.5 \pm 1.8.$$
$$Ce.M.: \quad 15.2 \pm 1.0, \; 2.3 \pm 0.6, \quad 8.9 \pm 1.3.$$
$$V.c.e.: \quad 16.4 \pm 1.2, \; 1.9 \pm 0.7, \; 15.1 \pm 1.4.$$

In Tables 3 to 7 the central letters refer to the method for siting
the lesion, R meaning recording, S stimulation and A anatomical co-
ordinates. The expected anatomical sites, derived from the atlas, are
to the left of this central column and the results to the right, with the
period of follow-up, or, if the improvement was temporary, its duration.
Where two or more nuclei are affected by a single lesion they are underlined. As seen already, there is no obvious correlation between method
of lesion siting and results.

In general, there was good agreement between the expected anatomical sites and recording, but for three lesions the finding of evoked
limb responses suggested that a lesion expected to be in V.im. also

included part of V.c.e., and for one lesion the finding of evoked responses from the head suggested that V.c.i. was included as well as V.c.e. This assumes that limb evoked responses do not occur in V.im., or head responses in V.c.e.; in one instance, head responses may have occurred in V.c.p.c. These five lesions are marked by an asterisk. In only two instances (denoted by a dagger), did a lack of appropriate evoked responses, despite thorough testing, suggest that lesions judged from the atlas as likely to include one of the sensory relay nuclei (V.c.i.) probably did not.

The outcome in essential tremor (Table 3) was gratifying, since it was abolished in all cases, and sometimes a single lesion probably in V.i.m. was enough. Other authors (Mundinger et al. 1970, Cooper 1969, Obrador

Table 3. *Essential Tremor*

		Simple		
(1)	L	Vim *	RS	Abolished—1 year
(2)	L	Vce Vcpc *	RS	Abolished—5 years
	R	Vim Vce	S	
(3)	L	Vce Vim	S	Abolished—5 years
		Associated with Spasmodic Torticollis		
(1)	R	CI Vce	S	Abolished—7 years
	L	Vim	S	
(2)	L	CeM Vim * Vim	A	Abolished—3 months
	R	Vim Vci Cem †	A	

and Dierssen 1965) have also published good results. Our third case was surprisingly relieved of tremor after two small lesions on one side. An identical tremor may occur with spasmodic torticollis and two cases were relieved of all abnormal movements by stereotaxis. It was the experience of Laitinen and Johansson (1966) that the results of stereotaxis are better in those with tremor and torticollis than in those with torticollis alone.

Table 4 concerns those with severe intention tremor and the results are less satisfactory than for essential tremor, possibly because the patients were initially more disabled. In the third case, a lesion in or near V.im. abolished the tremor on one side but the effect of the lesion on the other side was temporary. A second attempt caused hemiplegia, probably owing to the patient's insistence on general anaesthesia. In other cases, the tremor was either improved or the relief was temporary. In disseminated sclerosis we insist on operating in a quiescent phase, under cover of ACTH.

In spasmodic torticollis (Table 5), three lesions are first made on one side, the first two being sited physiologically, as for the tremor cases, and the third is then placed in the centro-medianum which has 100% probability in the atlas. Results of other surgeons have been

Table 4. *Intention Tremor*

Aetiology Uncertain

(1)	R	Vim Vce	R	Greatly improved—6 months
(2)	L	Vim Vce Vcpc Vce	RS	Temporary improvement— 3 months
(3)	L	1 Vim Vce Vci	R	Temporary improvement (hemianaesthesia)
		2 Vim	A	Hemiplegia
	R	Vim	S	Abolished—2 years

Due to Disseminated Sclerosis

(1)	R	Vim	S	Temporary improvement— 6 months
(2)	R	Vce Vim	R	Improved—2 years
(3)	L	Vim Vce Vci Oe Vim	RS	Improved—1 year
(4)	L	Vim	S	Greatly improved—3 years

Table 5. *Spasmodic Torticollis or Retrocollis*

(1)	L	Vim Vci Vce † CeM CNR	RS	Temporary—1 year
	R	CI Oe CeM Vce	RS	
(2)	L	Vim Oe CNR CeM Vim	R	Temporary—3 months
	R	Vim Oe Vce CeM	S	
(3)	L	Vim CeM Vim Oe	S	Temporary—14 months
	R	Vce	RS	
(4)	L	Vim Vce CeM	RS	Abolished—5 years
	R	Vim	S	
(5)	L	Vim CeM Vce CI Oe Vim	S	Abolished—7 years
	R	CI Vim Vce	S	
(6)	L	Vim Vce Vci CNR CeM	R	Abolished—4 years

variable. They have stressed the importance of bilateral lesions, though Hassler and Dieckmann (1970) have recently relieved torticollis by lesions in ventro-oralis internus and the field of Forel (H 1) on one side. Of our patients, only one, shown at the bottom of Table 5, had lasting abolition after unilateral thalamotomy. In this patient, possible record-ing-electrode slippage led to one lesion being made where the atlas indicated the capsule of the red nucleus (C.N.R.). He has a persistent postural tremor of the right hand but is delighted to be rid of the abnormal neck movements. In the other five patients, unilateral lesions did not stop the abnormal movements (though in the two cases of retrocollis they changed the movement to torticollis to the side opposite the lesions).

Table 6. *Torsion Dystonia*

Unilateral

(1)	L	Vce CI			RS	Greatly improved—5 years
(2)	R	Vce Vci VcP Vce Vim			RS	Improved—3 years
		Field of Forel Vce				
(3)	R	Vim*			R	Slightly improved—2 months

Generalized and associated with Spasmodic Torticollis

(1)	L	Vce* Vim Vce			R	Slightly improved—3 years
	R	Vim Vim Vci			S	
		CeM Vci Oe Field of Forel				

Table 7. *Hemiballismus*

| (1) | L | Vim Vce Vci CeM | | | R | Abolished |
| | | Vim | | | | |

Huntington's Chorea

(1)	L	Oe Vim	A	Relief of tremor
	R	CI	S	
(2)	L	Vce Oe Vim Vim	S	Relief of tremor
	R	Oe Vim CeM	A	

Although we were prepared to make the same three lesions in the other thalamus, the first or second lesion sometimes stopped the movement. Unfortunately cessation was only temporary in three cases.

All the patients with bilateral lesions have some degree of persisting dysarthria. Cooper (1969), who makes large bilateral lesions, reported a 70% success rate and a 20% risk of persisting dysarthria. It must be stated, however, that although our lesions are smaller, they are in discrete regions and may exert a greater functional effect. The only other side-effect was a short-lasting hemiparesis in the first and second cases who had a rather low-lying lesion probably affecting the C.N.R.

Table 6 gives the results in torsion dystonia, by which we mean a disturbance of muscle tone in which an abnormal posture is maintained for a considerable time. We have no case of dystonia musculorum deformans because all had evidence of neurological damage before the abnormal movement began. In one it followed head injury, in another encephalitis, and in two was apparently related to birth trauma. Thus it is impossible to compare with the large series of Cooper (1969) including only cases of dystonia musculorum deformans. All our patients improved to a certain extent, but the result was really gratifying in just two of those with unilateral dystonia.

We have a single case of hemiballismus (Table 7), in whom relief was complete although he now has mild tremor of the outstretched arm; and two cases of Huntington's chorea in whom the movements were markedly improved although they now show progressive mental deterioration as expected. We operate on patients with this disease only when there is no evidence of dementia, where the movements are restricted to the limbs and there is no serious disturbance of balance.

In conclusion, we find that small lesions in the somatic relay nuclei may be effective, although analysis of operations in which one or more of the lesions included a zone giving evoked responses from stretching of limb muscles reveals that the outcome is not consistently different from cases in which this has not been an established fact. We try to avoid the posterior part of V.c.e. and V.c.i., as well as ventro-caudalis parvocellularis and portae, for fear of producing permanent paraesthesiae. Some authors have restricted their lesions to the more anterior structures such as V.im., the oral ventral nuclei, the pallido-fugal pathways to the thalamus or the capsule itself, and found them effective. We also consider V.im. to be an effective target. However, we would like to conclude that in the circuitry necessary for the maintenance of involuntary movements of various types there may be an afferent component, namely the anterior part of the relay nuclei, where lesions may be beneficial.

Abbreviations Not Explained in Text

V.c.p.c. = Ventro-caudalis parvo-cellularis.
C.I.   = internal capsule.
O.e.   = oralis externus.
V.c.P.   = ventro-caudalis portae.

Acknowledgements

We wish to thank Mr. Drury of the Middlesex Hospital for his assistance with the tables; also Dr. Hewer and the Department of Clinical Measurement of the Middlesex Hospital and Miss Miller of the EEG Department, Oldchurch Hospital, for much assistance with the recordings.

References

1. Andrew, J., Rudolf, N. de M. (1972), Micro-electrode recordings in the human thalamus during stereotaxic surgery. In "Interdisciplinary Investigation of the Brain", p. 53—72. London and New York: Plenum Press.
2. — — (1973), Somatic representation in the human thalamus. J. Neurol. Neurosurg. Psychiat. *36,* 154.
3. — Watkins, S. (1969), A stereotaxic atlas of the human thalamus and adjacent structures. A variability study. Baltimore: Williams and Wilkins Co.
4. Cooper, I. S. (1969), Involuntary movement disorders. Hoeber Medical Division. New York: Harper and Row.
5. Hassler, R., Dieckmann, G. (1970), Stereotactic treatment of different kinds of spasmodic torticollis. 4th Symp. Int. Soc. Res. Stereoencephalotomy, New York, 1969. Confin. Neurol. *32,* 135—143.
6. Laitinen, L., Johannsson, G. G. (1966), Stereotaxic treatment of hyperkinesia. Nordisk Medicin *75,* 676—679.
7. Marshall, J. (1968), Handbook of clinical neurology (ed. P. J. Vinken and G. W. Bruyn) *6,* 809. Amsterdam: North American Publishing Co.
8. Mundinger, F., Riechert, T., Disselhoff, J. (1970), Long term results of stereotaxic operations on extrapyramidal hyperkinesias (excluding Parkinsonism). 4th Symp. Int. Soc. Res. Stereoencephalotomy, New York, 1969. Confin. Neurol. *32,* 71—78.
9. Obrador, S., Dierssen, G. (1965), Observations on the treatment of intentional and postural tremor by subcortical stereotaxic lesions. 2nd Int. Symp. Stereoencephalotomy, Copenhagen, 1965. Confin. Neurol. *26,* 250—253.
10. Rudolf, N. de M. (1969), Somatic representation in the human thalamus. EEG clin. Neurophysiol. *27,* 709.

Authors' address: Dr. N. de M. Rudolf, Department of Clinical Neurophysiology, Charing Cross Hospital, London, W 6 8RF, England.

Acta Neurochirurgica, Suppl. 21, 49—55 (1974)
© by Springer-Verlag 1974

Department of Neurosurgery, University of Groningen, The Netherlands

Stereotaxic Operations in Cases of Hereditary and Intention Tremor

J. van Manen

Since 1958 in our department we have examined approximately 900 cases of Parkinson's disease. Parkinsonism and related disorders with tremor as a main symptom, among these patients we saw 71 cases in which the tremor was more obvious during voluntary movement or in an active posture than at rest. Most of these showed at rest no tremor at all. No rigidity was found nor cogwheel phenomenon. These syndromes are extensively discussed by McDonald Critchley (1949) and more recently by E. Critchley (1972), whilst the mechanisms of tremors and the therapeutic possibilities have been studied by Poirier (1970).

The diagnosis of multiple sclerosis with intention tremor was made in 8 cases. Two cases had a clear post-traumatic, post-concussional etiology. In one case the diagnosis of an ill-defined spinocerebellar degeneration had to be made because of disturbance of gait. Dyssynergia cerebellaris myoclonica was diagnosed in one case because of a severe intention tremor-like dyskinesia, that did not disappear completely at rest, and associated with epileptic fits of some years duration.

The diagnosis of essential tremor was made in 7 monosymptomatic tremor cases without any sign of Parkinsonism and no hereditary component as far as the anamnesis concerned. Only one of these showed purely rest tremor, disappearing when the hands were outstretched or during intentional movements. The diagnosis of hereditary tremor was made in 52 cases and was based on the history and the presence of tremor in action as the only complaint and symptom (Table 1).

The incidence of this disease of a more or less serious degree can be estimated at $\frac{1}{2}$–1 per 10,000 population in comparison with the figures of 1 or 2 per 1000 for Parkinson's disease. The age at which the first symptoms appeared, sex, duration of illness and the data about heredity of these cases have been studied (Table 2). Heredity seems to be of a dominant type as also has been suggested by other authors (Critchley

J. van Manen:

1949). Hereditary factors were found in 20–25% in our 830 cases of
Parkinson's disease or Parkinsonism. The tremor usually appeared
during action that is of the intention type, absent at rest and exaggerated
by emotional stress. Except for handling buttons, feeding and writing
these patients were not seriously incapacitated by their tremor. The

Table 1. *Our Material*

± 900 cases	Parkinson's disease, Parkinsonism and related disorders
± 830 cases	Parkinson's disease and Parkinsonism (1–2/1000)
71 cases	Postural and intention tremor
52 cases	Hereditary tremor (½–1/10,000)
9 cases	Essential tremor (1 Ramsay Hunt syndrome?)
	(1 Cerebellar degeneration?)
2 cases	Posttraumatic tremor
8 cases	Sclerosis multiplex

Table 2. *Hereditary Tremor*

	52 cases	
	Female 17	Male 35
First complaints	0–20 years	17 cases
	21–44 years	12 cases
	45–60 years	18 cases
	61–72 years	5 cases
Mean duration of illness	11 years	
Hereditary factors		
One parent ± brothers/sisters		44
One grandparent		5
Brothers/sisters of parents/cousins		3
		52

time of onset and distribution of the symptoms have also been analysed
(Table 3). In two cases a torticollis also existed. One patient should
perhaps be diagnosed as a Roussy-Levy syndrome because of signs of
neurogenic muscular atrophy (Table 4).

The tremor frequency was assessed in a number of cases and compared with the frequency in Parkinson's disease. Acceleration trans-
ducers and surface electromyography were used. We did not find
frequencies of more than 8 c/sec contrary to the statement of McDonald

Critchley (1949) and E. Critchley (1972). No clear differences between the several age groups were found so that the findings of Marshall (1962) regarding the association with physiological tremor could not be confir-

Table 3. *Hereditary Tremor* (52 cases)

Complaints

Tremor at rest ⟨ action	8 cases	
Attitude or action tremor of the hand	43 cases	
Tremor capitis	6 cases	

Symptoms

Tremor upper extremities	52 cases	⎡ slight	11
Unilateral	5 cases	⎪ moderate	29
Bilateral	47 cases	⎣ serious	13
Tremor lower extremities	25 cases	⎡ slight	21
		⎣ moderate	4
Tremor capitis	30 cases	⎡ slight	19
		⎪ moderate	8
		⎣ serious	3
Torticollis	2 cases	(combined with tremor capitis)	
Neurogenic muscular atrophy	1 case		
No dysarthria, nystagmus nor ataxia			

Table 4. *Tremor Frequency*

Hereditary tremor	(17 cases)	6.1 c/s	(attitude)	(irregular)
Parkinson's disease	(11 cases)	4.5 c/s	(at rest)	(regular)
		5.1 c/s	(attitude)	
Sclerosis multiplex and coarse intention tremor	(3 cases)	3–4 c/s		

Hereditary tremor (mean frequencies)

0–20 y	31–40 y	41–50 y	51–60 y	61–70 y	71–80 y
(1 case)	(3 cases)	(3 cases)	(2 cases)	(7 cases)	(1 case)
7	6.2	6.8	6	5.5	6.5

Range: 4.5–8 c/s

med. Postural tremor in these cases was measured with the arms outstretched. The mean frequency is higher than the mean frequency in Parkinson's disease, but in hereditary tremor a larger range of frequencies was found.

4*

In cases of Parkinson's disease the tremor seemed to be accelerated
somewhat with sustained posture after the fingernose test. The significance of these figures is not yet determined.

In the group of patients with hereditary and essential tremor several
kinds of medical treatment were investigated with poor results
(Table 5). Following the work of Sigwald and Dereux (1956) we tried
the effect of large doses of vitamin B 6 (pyridoxine 3×750 mg) for

Table 5. *Medical Therapy*

Barbiturates		zw + (3×)	0 (9×)	
Tranquillisers	+ (2×)	zw + (1×)	0 (16×)	
Antihistamines		zw + (1×)	0 (11×)	
Pyridoxine		zw + (1×)	0 (9×)	
Amantadine			0 (11×)	— (1×)
L-Dopa			0 (5×)	

Table 6. *Results of Operations* (V.L.)

Multiple sclerosis	(unilat.)	4 cases
Complete recurrence of tremor after some weeks of months		2 cases
Very slight improvement		2 cases
Slight general derioration		3 cases
Post-traumatic tremor	(unilat.)	2 cases
No improvement		1 case
Moderate improvement and slight aggravation of gait disturbances		1 case (7 years)

4 weeks and found a slight in one and a negative effect in the other
cases. Most patients react favourably for a short time with alcohol.
Amantadine, ·which releases dopamine, has been used over the past
two years as an reliable aid in the differential diagnosis of these diseases
with Parkinsonism. This saves time and discomfort for patients, if there
is no response to Amantadine we do not give L-Dopa. In this connection
it is perhaps worthwhile mentioning that micrographic handwriting is
a reliable sign leading to the diagnosis of Parkinsonism.

29 patients were operated upon. In all cases lesions in the ventro-
lateral nucleus of the thalamus were made with their centre 14 to 15 mm
behind the foramen of Monro, 2 mm above the FM-CP line and 14 to
15 mm lateral to the midline. Usually the lesion was enlarged in the
direction of the thalamic fasciculus. Thermo-coagulation lesions in and

2 mm below the target point at 70–80 °C were made of a diameter
of 6–8 mm. No lesions were made deeper or more medial in the fields
of Forel or more anterior in the thalamus as suggested by Bertrand
et al. (1968). There was no mortality. At the end of the operation, the

Table 7. *Results of Operations*

Hereditary and essential tremor	23 cases
Unilateral operations	18 cases
Bilateral operations	5 cases
Mean duration of illness	24 years
Mean age	54 years

10–30 years	31–45 years	46–55 years	56–65 years	66–72 years
1	6	3	8	5

Tremor	serious or moderate → zero	9 cases
	serious or moderate → slight	13 cases
	serious → moderate	1 case

complete recurrence after 4 years 1 case (3 years 90% result)

Follow-up 3 months—8 years
mean   2 years

Table 8. *Side-Effects*

		unilat. op.	bilat. op.
Gait disturbances	(slight)	3	1
	(serious)	1	–
Tendency to fall	(slight)	1	–
Lack of dexterity		3	–
Dysarthria	(slight)	2	3

tremor was always completely abolished, but when recurrences took
place they did so in the first two months after operation.

The results of the operations after 3 months or later for cases of
multiple sclerosis and post-traumatic tremor have been analysed and in
general the outcome is very poor (Table 6). The operations for hereditary
and essential tremor were much more rewarding (Table 7). Side-effects
of the operations were disturbances of gait, tendency to fall to the side
contralateral to the lesion and dysarthria (Table 8). A number of patients

complained in the first weeks of a lack of dexterity of the hand on the side operated without demonstrable sensory disturbances or distinct paresis. In three cases this complaint persisted unless physiotherapy was used regularly. The patients were interviewed about their assessment of the result of the operation by the surgeon and psychologist (Table 9). This gave a less satisfactory result than was shown by the absence of tremor alone. Bilateral operations give better results overall in respect

Table 9. *Judgement of Patient* (23 cases)

	unilat. op.	bilat. op.
Completely satisfied	5	2
Note quite satisfied because of side-effects	3	–
Not quite satisfied because of remaining tremor	2	1
Not quite satisfied because of other symptoms (e.g. torticollis)	1	1
Not quite satisfied because of tremor on the second side or tremor capitis	5	–
Very much dissatisfied because of recurrence of tremor	1	–
Very much dissatisfied because of side-effects	–	2

of limb function, but there is the danger of side effects such as dysarthria and postural instability. Tremor of the head usually persists to some extent.

Based on these results we would agree with other authors (Guiot et al. 1960, Bertrand et al. 1969) that hereditary and essential tremor can be relieved satisfactory by operation.

However, taking into account the assessment of our treated patients the indication for operation must be made carefully particularly as many of them show no or very little disability and are mainly handicapped by tremor produced by emotional stress.

Also slightside effects therefore must be kept to a minimum if operation is to be useful.

References

1. Critchley, McDonald (1949), Observations on essential (heredofamilial) tremor. Brain 72, 2, 113—139.
2. Sigwald, J., Bouttier, D., Piot, Cl., Hebert, H., Dereux, J. (1956), Le tremblement idiopathique. Action parfois remarquable de fortes doses de pyridoxine. Rev. Neurol. 94, 406—408.

3. Guiot, G., Brion, S., Fardeau, M., Bettaieb, A., Molina, P. (1960), Dyski-
   nésie volitionnelle d'attitude sumprimée par la coagulation thalamo-
   capsulaire. Rev. Neurol. *102*, 220—229.
4. Marshall, J. (1962), Observations on essential tremor. J. Neurol. Neurosurg. Psychiat. *25*, 122—126.
5. Bertrand, Cl., Hardy, J., Molina-Negro, P., Martinez, S. N. (1968), Optimum physiological target for the arrest of tremor. Third Symposium
   on Parkinson's Disease, 251—258. Edinburgh and London: E. & S.
   Livingstone Ltd.
6. — — — (1969), Tremor of attitude. Confin. Neurol. *31*, 37—41.
7. Poirier, L. J. (1970), Recent views on tremors and their treatment.
   Modern trends in Neurology *5*, 80—96. Ed. by D. Williams. London:
   Butterworths.
8. Critchley, E. (1972), Clinical manifestations of essential tremor. J.
   Neurol. Neurosurg. Psychiat. *35*, 365—373.

Author's address: J. van Manen, M.D., Oude Steeg 3, Glimmen (Gr),
The Netherlands.

Acta Neurochirurgica, Suppl. 21, 57—63 (1974)
© by Springer-Verlag 1974

Neurosurgical Clinic, Division for Stereotaxy, University of Cologne,
Federal Republic of Germany

Contributions to the Pathogenesis of Parinaud's Syndrome. Vertical Gaze Paralysis Following Bilateral Stereotaxic Lesion in the Interstitial Nucleus Region

K. Nittner and I. N. Petrovici

With 4 Figures

In 1886, Parinaud described a case of paralysis of the upward gaze in patients with lesions in the upper midbrain. The most frequent cause of this syndrome is a tumour (pinealoma) compressing the quadrigeminal plate. Less commonly, vascular disease and occasionally infection (encephalitis) may yield such a clinical picture. Although as early as 1905 Spiller demonstrated that the superior colliculi play no significant role in eye movements, especially in the vertical plane, some authors persist in attributing a faulty upward gaze in the case of lesions situated in the region of the tectum to involvement of the superior colliculus. This was disproved by Dereux (1926), Angelergues et al. (1957), and Christoff et al. (1962) in man, by Sager and Voiculescu (1950) in the cat and by Pasik and Pasik (1964) and Pasik et al. (1966) in the monkey.

Based on extensive studies of Hess on cats, Hassler (1960) summarized the head and eye movements as follows:—the rotatory movement around the longitudinal axis occurs towards the side of the stimulation by stimulating the interstitial nucleus; the raising movement is elicited by stimulation of the prestitial nucleus, the descending fibers of which form the medial portion of the medial longitudinal fasciculus; the downward movement is produced by stimulation of the precommissural nucleus, the descending fibers of which form the lateral area of the medial longitudinal fasciculus.

In man, the prestitial nucleus cannot be separated from the interstitial nucleus. Most authors consider that upward gaze weakness is due to bilateral lesions in the pretectum (Bender 1969), or a single one in the mid-portion of the posterior commissure (Sager and Voiculescu 1950). As a rule, patients manifesting defects in vertical eye movements show no lesion in the colliculi; conversely, lesions of the colliculi *per se* do not interfere with eye movements. Yet the fact must be stressed that in pathological cases in man we generally have to do with destructive or diffuse inflammatory lesions, it being impossible to state exactly

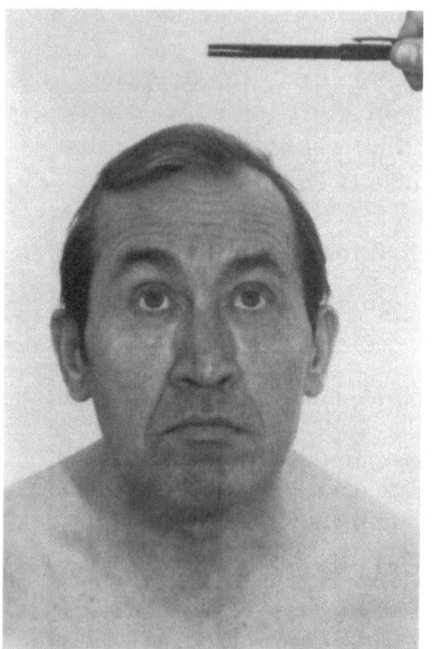 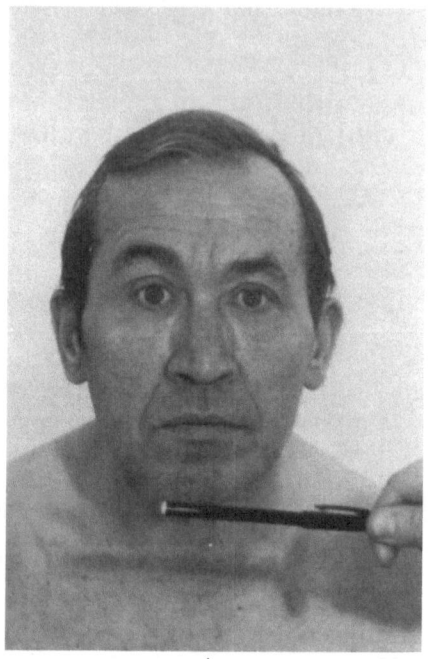

a   b

Fig. 1

which anatomical formations are involved in producing vertical eye movements. Experiments in animals are not always superposable with the observations made in regard to man.

That is why we considered it to be of interest to present our observation in which stereotaxic lesions restricted to a definite anatomical area have induced the appearance of a vertical paralysis of the gaze.

Sano et al. (1967, 1970) have shown that electric stimulation in the interstitial nucleus of Cajal or its adjacent area elicited marked EMG discharges and contraction of the bilateral posterior neck muscles accompanied by retroflexion of the neck. On the basis of these findings the authors proposed and performed the stereotaxic coagulation of this region in cases of retrocollis, whereby good results were reported.

We performed this operation in 4 patients, in three of whom it was unilateral only, while in one case a bilateral operation was performed. Among our cases with unilateral lesions, a patient developed postoperative paralysis of convergence which, however, subsided within a few weeks.

The case in which coagulation of the region of the interstitial nucleus was performed bilaterally forms the object of this communication.

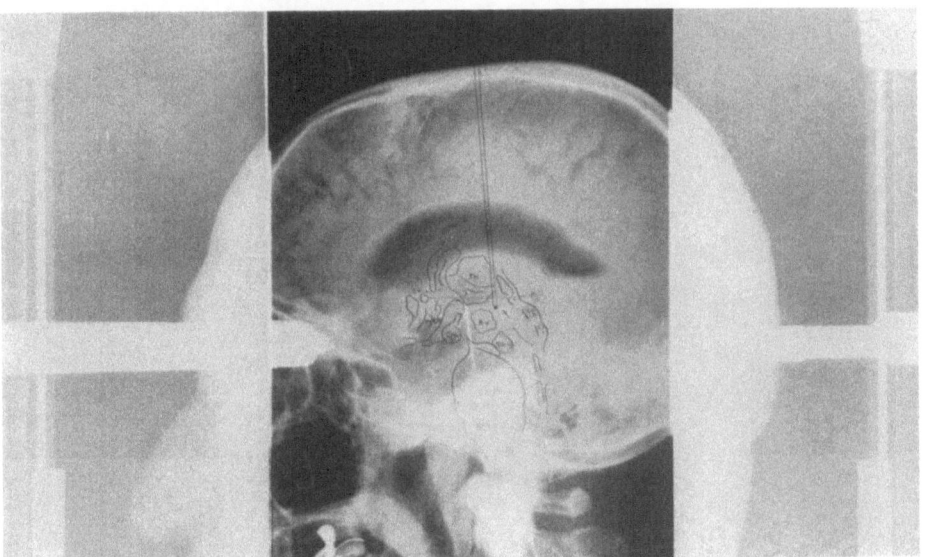

Fig. 2

The patient in question, a male aged 56, had suffered from retrocollis for 4 years. Stereotaxic coagulation was effected bilaterally in the course of a single operation. The coordinates of the target points were as follows: 9 mm posterior to the midpoint of the intercommissural line, 3 mm inferior to the intercommissural line, and 2 mm lateral to the mid-saggital plane. Electric stimulations (2 mA, 1 c/s and 5 msec pulse duration) brought about synchronous contractions in the muscles of the neck on the same side, while at 4 mA contractions were noticed also on the opposite side. No movements of the eye balls were observed. Electrocoagulation was first performed on the right side, there being no noticeable effects with regard to ocular movements. The electrode was then directed to the target point on the left side. While introducing the electrode no disturbances in ocular movements were noticed that might be due to a mechanical lesion. Towards the end of coagulation

on the left side the onset of a paralysis of the vertical eye movements
was noticed. Careful postoperative examination displayed an additional
lateral paresis of the gaze to the left and paralysis of convergence.
Subsequently, lateral paresis of the gaze subsided whereas paralysis
of the vertical eye movements as well as paralysis of the convergence
persisted unaltered (Figs. 1 a and b). The retrocollis was only slightly

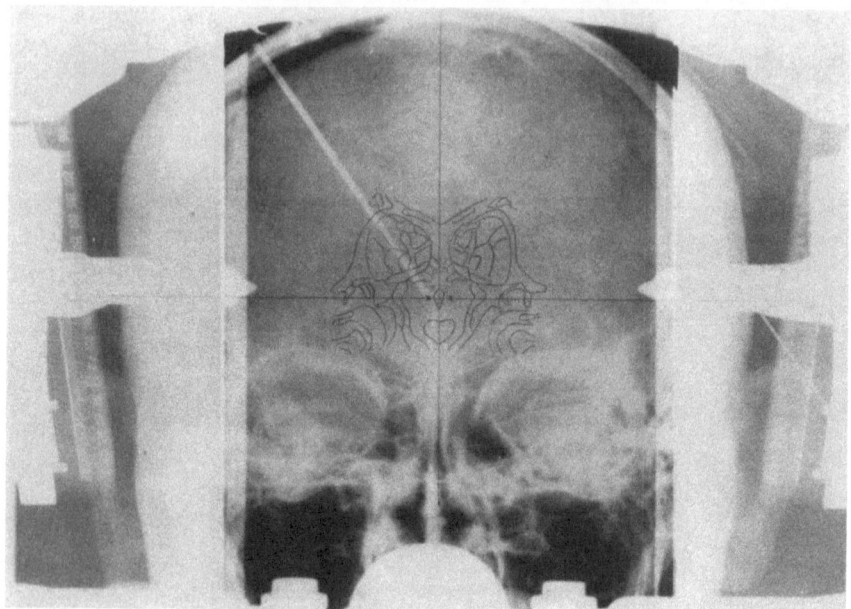

Fig. 3

improved a largely confined to a better posture of the head. No other
neurological deficit or alteration of consciousness were noticed.

Discussion

To the best of our knowledge our case represents a unique observation
in the literature, namely vertical paralysis of the gaze appearing in man
under quasi-experimental conditions consequent on lesions confined to
a specific zone of the midbrain. Although we are lacking the pathological
control, close examination of the radiological pictures and of the position
of the electrode permits us to affirm that the stereotaxic lesions were
performed in the area of the interstitial nucleus.

The direction of the electrode shows that a mechanical lesion of the
superior colliculi was impossible so that our case furnishes an additional

argument in support of the belief that these formations play no role whatever in vertical eye movements (Fig. 2). We cannot, however, exclude a concomitant lesion of the pretectal area, at any rate on the right side (Fig. 3). It is true that the appearance of ocular paralysis was observed by us only after we had performed the second coagulation on the opposite aspect. Yet the production of a lesion of the pretectal

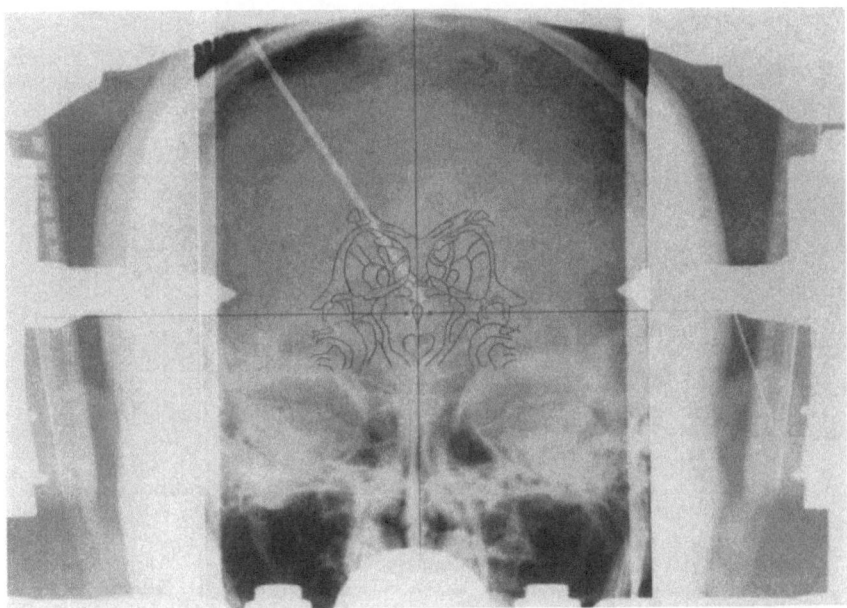

Fig. 4

area in both aspects cannot be excluded, as the stereotaxic lesion may be estimated at 3–4 mm in diameter and seeing that the area of the pretectum-posterior commissure is so small (Fig. 4).

As shown also by experiments in animals, our observation in man demonstrates the necessity of a bilateral lesion or of a lesion crossing the mid-line for the appearance of vertical paralysis of the gaze.

In the area of the pretectum-interstitial nucleus-posterior commissure verticogire fibers are believed to act as a relay in a thalamic-cortical system for the movements of the head and eyes in every direction of space. This area is tonically active as subsequent circumscribed coagulation of stimulation points abolish the stimulation effects and give rise to mirror image position of the head and the eyes. It therefore seems likely that the formations responsible for the movements of the head and those responsible for ocular movements may be different although the vertical movements of the head and eyes—as also the lateral movements—are conjugated forming part of a common neuro-physiological mechanism. Thus Sano et al. (1970) obtained an ameliora-tion in the posture of the head without reporting side-effects concerning the eye movements; in our case the complete and persisting paralysis of the vertical eye movements was merely associated with a slight improvement in the posture of the head.

In the course of subsequent operations the concomitant recording of the EMG of the neck muscles and of the electro-oculogram during electric stimulation may lead to the elucidation of this problem.

References

1. Angelergues, R., Ajuriaguerra, J. de, Hécaen, H. (1957), Paralysie de la verticalité du regard d'origine vasculaire ; étude anatomoclinique. Rev. Neurol. (Paris) *96*, 301—319.
2. Bender, M. B. (1969), Disorders of eye movements. In P. J. Vinken and G. W. Bruyn, edts.: Handbook of Clinical Neurology, Vol. 1, Disturbances of Nervous Function, pp. 574—630. Amsterdam: North-Holland Publ. Comp.
3. Christoff, N., Anderson, P., Bender, M. B. (1962), Clinico-pathologic study of associated vertical eye movements. Trans. Amer. neurol. Ass. *87*, 184—186.
4. Dereux, J. (1926), Paralysie verticale du regard (Syndrome de Pari-naud). Contribution à l'étude de la localisation de la lésion. Thèse, Paris.
5. Hassler, R. (1960), Thalamo-corticale Systeme der Körperhaltung und der Augenbewegungen. In D. B. Tower and J. P. Schadé, edts.: Structure and Function of the Cerebral Cortex, pp. 124—130. Amster-dam: Elsevier Publ. Comp.
6. Parinaud, H. (1883), Paralysies des mouvements associés des yeux. Arch. Neurol. Psychiat. (Chicago) *5*, 145—172.
7. — (1886), Paralysie de la convergence ; paralysie de divergence. Ann. Oculist. (Paris) *95*, 205.
8. Pasik, P., Pasik, T. (1964), Oculomotor functions in monkeys with lesions of the cerebrum and the superior colliculi. In M. B. Bender, ed.: The Oculomotor System, pp. 40—80. New York: Harper & Row.
9. — — Bender, M. B. (1966), The superior colliculi and eye movements. Arch. Neurol. (Chicago) *15*, 420—436.
10. Sager, O., Voiculescu, V. (1950), Etudes experimentales sur les voies cortico-oculogyres de verticalité. Folia psychiat. (Amst.) *53*, 394—407.
11. Sano, K., Yoshioka, M., Ogashiwa, M., Ishijima, B., Ohye, C., Sekino, H., Mayanagi, Y. (1967), Central mechanisms of neck movements in the human brain stem. Confin. Neurol. *29*, 107—111.
12. — — Mayanagi, Y., Sekino, H., Yoshimasu, N., Tsukamoto, Y. (1970), Stimulation and destruction of and around the interstitial nucleus of Cajal in man. In E. A. Spiegel and H. T. Wycis, edts.: Advances in Stereoencephalotomy, Vol. 5, pp. 118—125. Basel: S. Karger.

13. Spiller, W. G. (1905), The importance in clinical diagnosis of paralysis of associated movements of the eyeballs especially of upward and downward associated movements. J. nerv. ment. Dis. *32*, 417—530.

Authors' addresses: Prof. Dr. K. Nittner, Bachemer Straße 8, D-5000 Köln-Lindenthal, Federal Republic of Germany. Dr. I. N. Petrovici, Neurologische Klinik, Städtisches Krankenhaus, D-5000 Köln-Merheim, Federal Republic of Germany.

Acta Neurochirurgica, Suppl. 21, 65—70 (1974)
© by Springer-Verlag 1974

Neurosurgical and Otorhinolaryngological Departments, Salzburg, Austria

Vestibular Function before and after Thalamotomy

H. E. Diemath and N. Hibler

The problem of diencephalic disturbances of vestibular function is an old one. In connection with stereotactic surgery it has achieved new interest. One of us was concerned with this matter at the 4th Donau-symposium in Vienna whilst dealing with the origins of disturbances in gait and posture in Parkinsonian disease.

A vestibulothalamic tract has been predicted for a long time but was never prooved anatomically (Clara 1959). On the other hand there are a number of animal experiments showing nystagmogenic areas in the diencephalon (Cook-Cangiano-Pompeiano 1969, Montandon 1964, Spiegel-Szekely-Gildenberg 1964).

There are also reports on clinical investigations (Fisch-Siegfried 1965, Mamo-Dondey-Cophignon 1965, Metzel 1965, Veronese-Mingrino 1963) showing pre- and postoperative disturbances in vestibular function. Most of these reports are concerned with stereotactic lesions in the ventro-lateral area of the thalamus (VL). There are however no investigations comparing the effects of different targets in various diseases. Therefore we began to study these problems using different targets (Nucleus ventralis oralis, Nucleus dorsomedialis, Zona incerta, Columna fornicis) for therapeutic lesions in various diseases (Parkinsonism, Hemiparkinsonism, Tic, Pain and Epilepsy).

Methods

1. Examination of vestibular function. The routine method of the otorhinolaryngological department was used; the examination was done a few days preoperatively and 9 days postoperatively. In some cases follow up studies were made some weeks or months later.

The caloric response was tested by instilling 10 ml water at 18 °C, into the auditory canal for 10 seconds. A normal reaction was assumed when after a latency of 10–20 sec a horizontal rotary nystagmus of second degree directed to the opposite side was obtained during the period of 80 to 120 seconds. (Fränzel-Leuchbrille technique.)

Table 1

Nr.	Hemiparkinsonism	RR	PEG	EEG	Hearing	Vestibular Function	
						preop.	postop.
1	M. J. m. 60 ys left	130/80	n	n	n	+ left	− bilat.
2	H. J. m. 61 ys left	130/90	n	dysreg.	n	n	n
3	Ö. J. m. 47 ys right	120/70	Atr.	n	n	n	+ bilat.
4	S. E. f. 44 ys right	140/80	n	n	n	+ left	+ left
5	L. J. m. 35 ys right	120/80	n	n	n	− left	+ bilat.
6	W. J. m. 56 ys right	135/80	Atr.	n	Hypac.	n	irreg. Nyst.
7	B. J. f. 47 ys right	140/90	Atr.	n	n	irreg. Nyst.	

RR = bloodpressure, PEG = Pneumoencephalogram, EEG = Electroencephalogram, n = normal, Atr. = Atrophy, dysreg. = dysregularity without focal signs, + = increased sensibility, − = decreased sensibility, irreg. Nyst. = irregular Nystagmus.

2. Stereotactic operation. The Riechert-Mundinger apparatus was used. Targets were identified by X-ray control and electrical stimulation was done routinely. High frequency current of 0.25 MHz was used for making the lesion. With our electrode (Saitenelektrode of Mundinger) a final temperature of 80 °C was established with an average of 120 mA, 30 V and 30 sec duration. The calculated lesions are about 200 mm³ in the nucleus ventralis oralis, about twice this size in the dorsomedial nucleus and about 40 mm³ in the zona incerta.

Results

Out of 10 patients with adequate postoperative follow-up 7 patients with Hemiparkinsonism are listed (Table 1). The other patients were

Table 2. *O. Josef 47 ys*

Caloric response: *Preoperative* 29. 11. 1971
                  10 ccm 18° water

	Latency	Amplitude	Duration
Right	10″	horiz. rotat. 2.°	84″
Left	12″	horiz. rotat. 2.°	86″

Caloric response: *Postoperative* 15. 12. 1971
                  10 ccm 18° water

	Latency	Amplitude	Duration
Right	6″	horiz. rotat. 3.°	122″
Left	5″	horiz. rotat. 3.°	130″

suffering from bilateral Parkinsonism (male 63 years, probable arteriosclerotic etiology), from intractable spinal pain (male 48 years) and from intractable facial tic (male 72 years).

In the patients with Hemiparkinsonism the side effect of the diencephalic lesion was determined. Out of these 7 patients normal vestibular function was found in 3, in two there was a diminished response (one ipsilateral one contralateral to the assumed diencephalic lesion) and one had contralateral increased response. In one patient there was an irregular nystagmus (Table 1).

After the stereotactic operation the vestibular function did not change in one patient with normal findings, in three patients the response had increased (two bilaterally and one ipsilateral to the lesion, Table 2).

In one patient the response decreased bilaterally (Table 3) and in two patients there was an irregular nystagmus.

There were no postoperative disturbances of gait or lateropulsion in the Hemiparkinsonian group.

One patient with bilateral Parkinsonism developed a slight hemiparesis with disturbance of gait postoperatively but without lateropulsion. His vestibular function was normal pre- and postoperatively.

Table 3. *M. Johann 60 ys*

Caloric response: *Preoperative* 5. 10. 1971
               10 ccm 18° water

	Latency	Amplitude	Duration
Right	15″	horiz. rotat. 2.°	105″
Left	7″	horiz. rotat. 2.°	130″

Caloric response: *Postoperative* 15. 10. 1971
               10 ccm 18° water

	Latency	Amplitude	Duration
Right	15″	horiz. rotat. 1.–2.°	85″
Left	13″	horiz. rotat. 1.–2.°	105″

Discussion

There are a number of reports on preoperative and postoperative changes in the caloric response of the vestibular system in patients with Parkinsonism. However these reported findings are quite different and indeed present opposite effects not only preoperatively but also following thalamotomy. Some authors (Fisch and Siegfried 1965) report preoperatively a small but significant difference in the caloric response according to the predominant central lesion, i.e. a predominance of a left nystagmus in a right central lesion. On the other hand there are reports (Veronese and Mingrino 1963) showing the nystagmus directed to the side of the diencephalic lesion.

In our opinion there is no doubt that at least a part of these different and opposite findings is due to the specific problem of testing vestibular function. Furthermore etiology, duration, and the actual state of the disease and even the emotional state of the patients at the time of examination (Mayczak 1970) may modify the caloric response.

During postoperative assessment it is important to keep in mind the well known capacity for cerebral compensation: different findings at different intervals after making the lesion (Barlow 1970). The preliminary results of our investigation indicate that there is no correlation between pre- and postoperative changes of vestibular function of patients with Parkinsonism. The same seems true for postoperative (stereotactic thalamotomy) findings in patients with other diseases.

Our further investigations on a greater number of patients will endeavour to elucidate the significance of associated disease, etiology, and other findings e.g. changes in bloodpressure, EEG, ECG, PEG, fundus of the eye etc. and the effect of different lesions within the thalamus.

Summary

1. In patients with Parkinsonism vestibular function (caloric response) may be disturbed preoperatively and postoperatively (stereotactic lesions in nucleus ventralis oralis, and zona incerta, 8 patients).

2. Postoperative changes were found also in patients with other diseases e.g. pain, tic (3 patients).

3. The type of change (increase or decrease of vestibular sensibility) and degree cannot be predicted.

4. These changes are not found in all patients neither preoperatively nor postoperatively.

5. In contradiction to other reports there was no correlation between disturbed vestibular function and lateropulsion.

6. There is no relationship between the results of operation (tremor, rigidity, pain, tic) and changes in vestibular function post-operatively.

7. Specific problems of the methodology (caloric response) and the possibility of the influence of other diseases have to be considered.

References

1. Barlow, J. S. (1970), Vestibular and non dominant parietal lobe disorders. (Two aspects of spatial disorientation in man.) Dis. Nerv. Syst. *31*, 667—673.
2. Clara, M. (1959), Das Nervensystem des Menschen, 3. Aufl., pp. 808. Leipzig: J. A. Barth.
3. Cook, W. A., Cangiano, A., Pompeiano, O. (1969), An electrical investigation of the efferent pathways from the vestibular nuclei. Arch. Ital. Biol. *107*, 235—274.
4. Diemath, H. E., Stereotaktische Behandlung von Gang- und Haltungsstörungen beim Parkinsonsyndrom. Kongreßband, 4. Donau-Symposium für Neurologie, Wien 6.—9. Oktober 1971, Verlag d. Wien. Med. Akad., in Druck.

5. Fisch, U., Siegfried, J. (1965), Prä- und postoperative Untersuchungen über die Vestibularisfunktion beim Parkinsonismus. Schweiz. Arch. Neurol. Psychiat. *96*, 286—305.
6. Mamo, H., Dondey, M., Cophignon, J., Pialoux, P., Fontelle, P., Houdart, R. (1965), Latéro-pulsion transitoire aú décours de coagulations sous-thalamiques et thalamiques chez des parkinsoniens. Rev. Neurol. *112*, 509—520.
7. Majczak, A. (1970), Kliniczne Badania elektrycznej reaktywnosci uladu przedsionkowego. Psychiat. pol. *4/5*, 523—530.
8. Metzel, E. (1965), Über die Störung des Raumsinnes beim Parkinson-Syndrom. Dtsch. med. Wschr. *90*, 1955—1957.
9. Montandon, P. (1964), Functional correlation between the diencephalic nystagmogenic area (DNA) and the vestibular nystagmogenic area (VNA). Acta oto-laryng., Suppl. 186.
10. Riechert, T., Mundinger, F. (1959), Beschreibung und Anwendung eines Zielgerätes für stereotaktische Hirnoperationen. 2. Modell. Acta neurochir. (Wien), Suppl. *3*, 308—337.
11. Spiegel, E. A., Szekely, E. G., Gildenberg, P. (1964), Vestibular projection to mesodiencephalic nuclei and basal ganglia. Fed. Proc. *23*, 415.
12. Veronese, A., Mingrino, S. (1963), Osservazioni sul comportamento della reflettivita vestibulare in soggetti parkinsoniani prima e dopo intervento di talamolisis (rilievi elettronistagmografici). G. Psichiat. Neuropat. *91*, 379—390.

Authors' address: Primarius Prof. Dr. H. E. Diemath, Traunstraße 31, A-5026 Salzburg, Austria.

Acta Neurochirurgica, Suppl. 21, 71—73 (1974)
© by Springer-Verlag 1974

Hôtel-Dieu Hospital, University of Montreal, Canada

Post-Stereotaxic Intracranial Hematomas

P. H. Crevier

As a corollary to Professor Gillingham's introduction, I would like to say a few words about an international survey on the occurrence of post-stereotaxic intracranial hematomas, their sites and evolution. It was conducted by the author in 1968 and 1969.

Those 70 neurosurgical centers reported some 21,000 stereotaxic operations performed between 1952 and 1967. Considering that only 53% of the stereotactic surgeons answered the questionnaire, one may infer that some 40,000 stereotaxic operations were performed during that 15 year period. Those 8 per thousand intracranial hematomas were diagnosed obviously either by surgery or by post-mortem. This figure appears to be conservative because it does not include the amount of intracranial hematomas which did not yield clinical signs or whose signs were interpreted as resulting from an infarction. Therefore, in order to facilitate the answers to the survey and increase their number, I did not ask for the amount of post-stereotaxic thrombosis, clinically diagnosed. 95 out of the 171 intracranial hematomas died, or 56%. If the figure 95 is related to the absolute amount of stereotaxic operations, we come to a proportion of 5 per thousand. It appears that most omit neurosurgeons have abandoned the practice of operating on those post-stereotaxic intracranial hematomas during the first ten days of their occurrence, unless death is pending due to severe signs of increased intracranial pressure.

If we leave out those last three hematomas (Table 4), we could use the term intracerebral instead of intracranial.

The two published series that I have studied and included in this survey represented some 3000 operations. The authors did consider the sequelae of surgical cerebro-vascular accidents other than hematomas, and I have abstracted the two following figures: a) Motor deficit secondary to a vascular trauma: 14 per thousand cases submitted to stereotaxy. b) 32% of those surviving the evacuation of their intracranial

Table 1. *Number of Letters Sent to Chiefs of Neuro-Surgical Centers where Stereotaxy is Performed*

Number of letters	131
Useful answers received	70 (53%)
Published series used	2

Table 2. *Occurrence of Hematomas and Deaths in Reference to the Number of Cerebral Stereotaxic Operations Reported*

Number of operations (circa 1952 until 1967) =	20,941
Number of intracranial hematomas	171 (8‰)
Deaths secondary to hematomas	95 (5‰)
Average % of hematomas in large series	1 to 3

Table 3. *Sites of those 171 Hematomas*

a) Intra-thalamic	65 (37%)
b) Sub-cortical	12 (7%)
c) Intracerebral: along trajectory of electrode(s) without further precision	66 (38%)

Table 4. *Sites of those 171 Hematomas*

d) Sub-dural	17 (10%)
e) Intra-ventricular	8 (5%)
f) Epidural	1 (0.5%)
g) Sub-arachnoid	2 (1.5%)

Table 5. *Other Sequelae*

Proportion of motor deficit secondary to a vascular trauma (other than hematomas)	14‰
Proportion of motor deficit surviving evacuation of hematomas	32%

hematoma suffered from an incapacitating muscular weakness due to the fact of course that most of the burr holes are made in the vicinity of the coronal suture.

Comments

a) Considering the methods used for the destruction of the target, this survey deals with all the standard ones:

1) Heat and cold, or electrocoagulation and cryoprobes.

2) Pure physical means like the leucotome and the radioactive substances.

3) The chemical ones including wax and alcohol to which is usually added a contrast substance.

b) Although 75% of the surgeons seem to use electrocoagulation, intracranial hematomas appear to occur with an equal frequency within each of those methods. Therefore, it seems that the blame has to be put mostly on the blunt action of the carrier, whether it be a needle, an electrode or any sort of metallic probe, crossing the gray substance of the cortex or of the basal ganglia.

c) The results of this survey seem to suggest that plain Roentgen films, AP and lateral, be taken some 12 to 18 hours after the termination of the procedure, whether pathological signs are present or not.

d) The results of this survey represent a random but probably quite a vivid recall of this type of complication in the experience of stereotaxic surgeons, since it was obvious that less than 25% of the surgeons had time to go through their whole pile of dossiers, carefully and thoroughly, patient by patient. None of us has time to do so.

e) The results of this survey will be published elsewhere with more details.

Author's identity: P. H. Crevier, Neurosurgeon, F.R.C.S.(c). Dipl. A.B. N.S., Hôtel-Dieu Hospital, University of Montreal, Canada.
Author's address: 3875 St.-Urbain, Suite 317, Montreal H2W 1V1, Canada.

Section II

Hind Brain and Spinal Stereotactic Procedures

Acta Neurochirurgica, Suppl. 21, 77—88 (1974)
© by Springer-Verlag 1974

Division of Neurological Surgery, Department of Surgery, Tulane University
School of Medicine, New Orleans, Louisiana, U.S.A.

Thalamotomy for Control of Chronic Pain*

D. E. Richardson

With 8 Figures

Introduction

For the past several years I have attempted to develop a stereotaxic
procedure at the level of the thalamus for control of chronic pain.
A stereotaxic operation has several theoretical advantages over older
procedures such as rhizotomy, tractotomy, and prefrontal lobotomy
for pain. Firstly, procedures at this level would control pain over the
entire contralateral half of the body and would not be limited to anatomical segments, which would be helpful in difficult areas of pain
control such as craniocervical pain. Secondly, stereotaxic procedures
can be performed easily under local anesthesia, obviating the use of
general anesthesia and prolonged open operations on patients who are
often debilitated with advanced cancer. Thirdly, on theoretical grounds,
at the level of the thalamus sensation should be segregated into its
different components of touch, proprioception, temperature, and pain;
allowing preferential destruction of pain in the conducting system without the associated loss of sensation of other types. Fourth, anatomical
separation from the motor and other systems reduce the complications
of weakness, ataxia, and incontinence, that are not uncommonly seen
after tractotomy in the spinal cord or brain stem. Lastly, it should
not have the destructive effect on personality associated with prefrontal
lobotomy.

The major deterrent to the development of a procedure at the level
of the thalamus for relief of pain has been the lack of knowledge regarding
the physiology of pain transmission above the lower brain stem. The

* Supported by the Cancer Association of Greater New Orleans, Grant
118–170.

demonstration of Bishop in 1959[1], that the chronic pain pathways were not carried to the primary relay nucleus in the ventral posterior lateralis and ventral posterior medialis nuclei of the thalamus has been borne out in many studies in both animals and humans since that time. The pain fibres apparently leave the spinothalamic tract at the level of the brain stem to enter the reticular formation and ascend in a multisynaptic fashion that can be traced anatomically as far as the intralamina nucleus of the thalamus using the Nauta staining technique for unmyelinated fibres as described by Mehler[12] in 1960, and Bowsher[3] in 1957. In man, less than 25% of the spinothalamic tract reaches the ventral posterior nucleus, and in the cat apparently few or no fibres reach this area[1, 13]. Above this level, the pathways become quite difficult to follow anatomically as well as electrophysiologically. Acquiring enough human material to be meaningful for different areas of the thalamus and subthalamus requires a large number of patients and anatomical correlation which has been difficult to obtain in our cases. The study of the pain pathway in lower animals is, of course, hindered by the fact that one is never sure whether the fibre tract being traced anatomically or the response measured electrophysiologically is actually related to pain. With these reservations in mind, I would like to discuss some of my observations both in animals and in the human and try to make certain correlations between the basic electrophysiological studies in the animals and our experience in the human.

Results

Initial stimulation studies were carried out during stereotaxic procedures on the thalamus in the VPL and VPM. The response to stimulation of the primary sensory relay nucleus of the thalamus in the human is one of paresthesias at very low voltage levels, usually less than one volt at threshold with increase in voltage causing rapidly increasing paresthesiae to the point the patient could not tolerate the paresthesiae any further, but usually without significant pain. Stimulation between 10 and 100 HZ at levels significant to produce comfortable paresthesiae caused relief from chronic pain that persisted for several minutes following cessation of stimulation. At low frequency rates and slightly higher levels of stimulation, tremor of the contralateral extremities was noted. At higher frequency rates, paresthesiae and reduction of pain is noted at high levels of stimulation with some report of numbness of contralateral face and extremities. Touch and pin prick testing of these areas, however, reveals no reported loss of perception of sensation. At high frequency rates, tonic contraction of muscles of the trunk and extremities contralaterally also occurs and interfered with testing and description of

sensory phenomenon since the patients reported drawing or tightness
of the contralateral extremities and chest on a muscular basis. Muscular
phenomena were always at slightly higher threshold levels than sensory
phenomena which allows some separation of stimulus effects.

The patient's response to small lesions placed in the primary sensory
nucleus of the thalamus was marked loss of proprioception and touch
sensation, but relatively little change in the perception of pain. The
patients usually reported that the pain was more severe than pre-

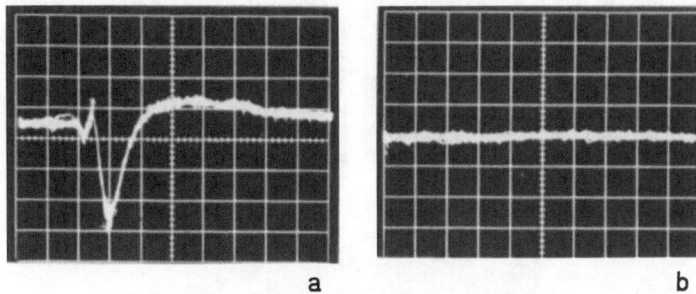

a   b

Fig. 1. Recording from nucleus ventral posterior lateralis before and after
section of dorsal column. Evoked responses in the cat is completely
abolished. AP = + 9.5; Lat. = 7; Ht. = O. 10 m sec/cm, 50 μv/cm.
Right leg stimulation. Cat Sl 19 (2–5). a pre-cardotomy, b post-dorsal
cordotomy

operatively and in addition to their pain they were disturbed by numbness
and sensory ataxia.

The evoked potential recordings made from the ventral posterior
nucleus in the cat revealed that short latency responses can be easily
obtained from electrical shock of the sciatic nerve and that if dorsal
chordotomy is carried out, this response is almost completely abolished
as seen in Fig. 1.

Our attention was next turned to the area just medial to the primary
sensory nucleus as suggested by Mark and Ervin[9] in some of their earlier
studies on this portion of the sensory thalamus based on the suggestion
of Bowsher[3]. Stimulation studies and lesions were produced in the area
of the center median and parafasicular nucleus. In the human, the
parafasicular nucleus is a rudimentary structure and the centre median
was primarily used as a target. Initially, 24 patients were operated
with stimulation followed by lesions in the centre median. Stimulation
of the centre median results in paresthesiae much as described in the
primary sensory nucleus, but less well localized and occurring at higher
threshold levels, usually 1–3 volts. As stimulation is gradually increased

in the area of the centre median, the patient complains of increasing
discomfort and then at a level several volts above threshold would
suddenly complain of severe painful paresthesiae involving the opposite
side of the body. Radiofrequency lesions in the centre median produced
relief of chronic pain over the contralateral half of the body and bilateral

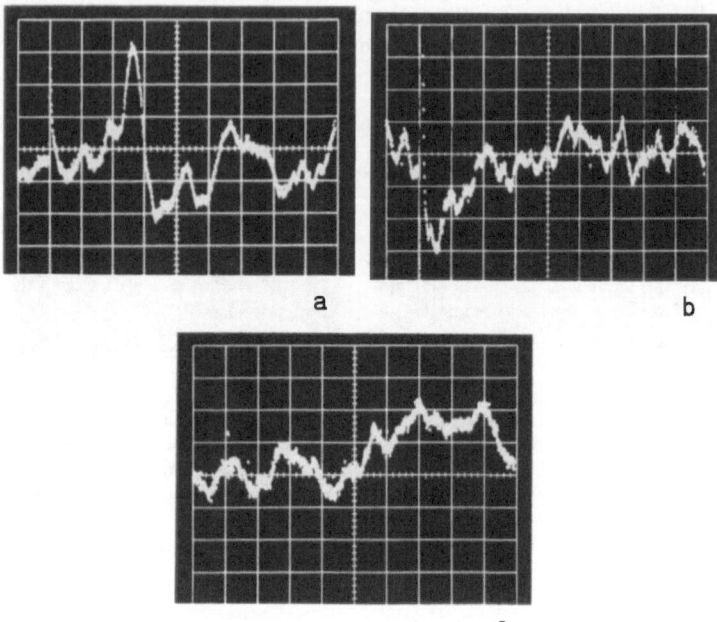

Fig. 2. Evoked response in centre median by somatosensory input showing
changes following section of dorsal columns. 25 m sec/div, 100 responses.
TP 93-2-10-11. a evoked response in left cm to right leg stimulation, b immediately after dorsal column section, c half hour after dorsal column
section

lesions would control bilateral pain of a chronic nature. Epicritic or
acute painful sensation was perceived normally and without loss of
localization or distortion following surgery. Sensory measurements
using focused heat lamp studies before and after surgery reveal no
difference in the threshold for acute painful stimuli. Painful experiences
in the patient following centre median lesions caused immediate pain
as would normally be expected, but when the well localized acute pain
response had subsided and would normally be replaced by a more
diffuse chronic pain, the pain simply subsides and no chronic pain
develops.

Electrophysiological studies carried out in cats reveal that evoked responses to sensory input could be easily obtained from the area of the centre median and parafasicularis nuclei following dorsal chordotomy as seen in Fig. 2. Following dorsal chordotomy, evoked responses still persistent in the area of the centre median can be abolished by ventral

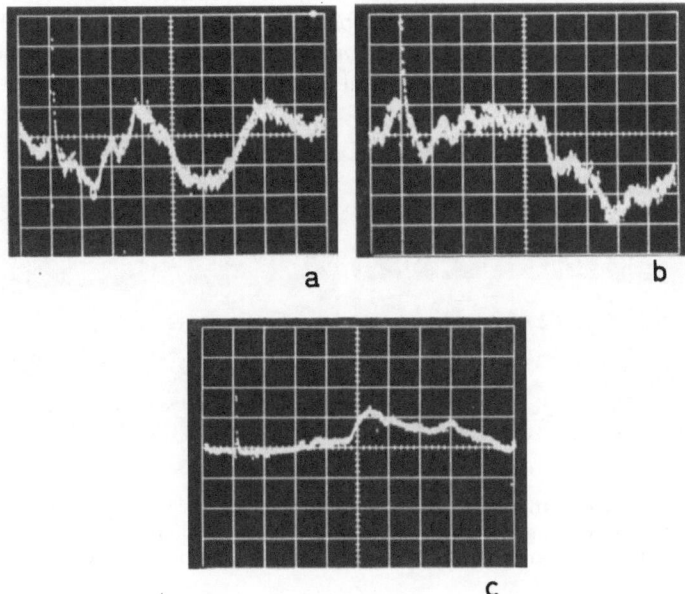

Fig. 3. Evoked response in pulvinar to somatosensory input reduced by dorsal column section, but markedly reduced by reticular formation lesion destroying paliospinothalamic pathways. 25 m sec/div, 100 responses. TP 93-pl-1-8-14. a evoked response in left pulvinar to right leg stimulation, b after dorsal column section, c after bilateral mesencephalic reticular formation lesion

lateral chordotomy. The pathway from the ventrolateral cord to the centre median was found to be abolished by producing bilateral lesions in the area of the brain stem reticular formation confirming Bowsher's anatomical and Collins' electrophysiological works[4, 6]. Collins has shown that unit recordings of cells in the centre median and reticular formation respond to somatosensory input by prolonged after discharge and has been able to correlate this prolonged after discharge of the centre median cells with peripheral stimuli only sufficient to produce firing of C fibres in the peripheral nerve[7]. Studies on humans have shown that C fibre stimulation in the peripheral nerve causes exquisite and severe pain which the patient will often not allow to be repeated[8].

The patients with lesions in the centre median have some minor abnormalities in personality, in that immediately following surgery they have a short period of euphoria. It has been difficult, clinically, to determine whether this euphoria is because the patient is relieved of his chronic unrelenting pain or whether it is a primary effect of the lesion in the thalamus. In any event, the euphoria subsides within 2–3 days in most cases, but relief of pain will persist for many months.

Only four patients have had stimulation studies of the dorsomedial nucleus and only one patient has had bilateral lesion production for pain

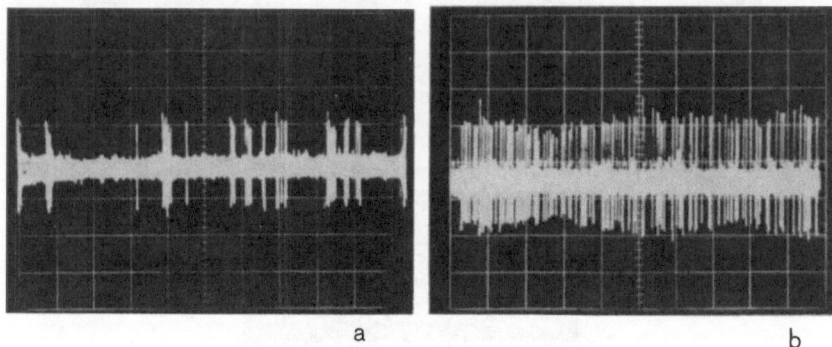

a   b

Fig. 4. Type I cell in pulvinar responding to C fiber input with prolonged after discharge lasting six minutes. Cat Sl 72-9-11, 500 m sec/cm. a resting firing pattern, b following burst stimulation to sciatic nerve

in this area. Stimulation at low levels usually produces no response, but increase of stimulation to 3 to 5 volts produces agitation and obvious discomfort without sensory phenomenon being reported. This response is somewhat similar to the response to cingulum stimulation that I have previously reported[15]. This stimulation is poorly understood by the patient and poorly described, but seems to be severe anxiety and agitation that is often denied following termination of the stimulation. The one bilaterally lesioned patient remained obtunded for several days and when recovered he reported his pain was unchanged. I have not been impressed enough with this area's relationship to pain transmission to carry out basic electrophysiological studies on the dorsomedial nucleus.

In the human thalamus, the centre median lies just medial to the ventral posterior medialis nucleus and the patients who have had lesions extending from the centre median into the medial portion of the VPM report sensory loss, both proprioception and touch and complain of upsetting numbness. In an attempt to reduce the incidence of objectionable sensory loss, the lesions were gradually moved posteriorly with similar results. It became obvious that lesions in the medial portion of the pulvinar caused a reduction of painful phenomenon similar to lesions in the centre median, that is, abolition of chronic pain without changes in acute pain perception[17], and has been carried out in 20 patients.

Stimulation of the medial pulvinar causes paresthesias much as does the centre median, but relatively better localized with higher threshold levels (1.5 to 4 volts), and when raised to several volts above threshold

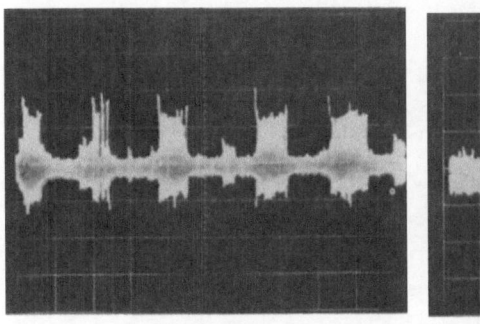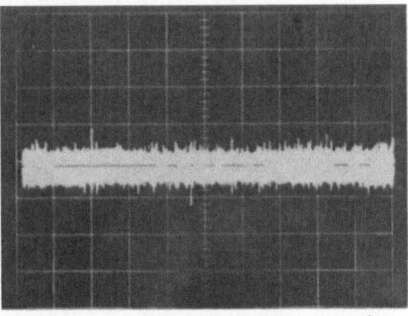

a   b

Fig. 5. Type II cell in pulvinar responding to C fiber input with inhibition of firing for six minutes. Cat Sl 73-9-10, 1 sec/cm. a resting pattern, b following burst stimulation to sciatic nerve

results in the onset of painful paresthesiae. The paresthesiae will often be localized to one segment of the body such as an arm, a leg, or the face. This is probably because the structure is larger in relation to the size of the stimulating electrode than the centre median.

Electrophysiological studies in the cat reveal that evoked responses from sensory input could be easily obtained by averaging techniques in the pulvinar as seen in Fig. 3, and that much like evoked responses in the centre median were reduced by dorsal chordotomy but not abolished unless dorsal chordotomy and ventral lateral chordotomy were carried out simultaneously. The reciprocal of this is also true. Lesions in the reticular formation reduced the evoked responses, but the addition of dorsal chordotomy was necessary to completely abolish the response[14, 16].

Extracellular microelectrode recording of single unit potentials in the pulvinar of the cat, which has been prepared with bilateral dorsal column section, reveal cells that respond to sensory input much as cells do in the centre median, with prolonged after discharge at levels of

stimulation calculated to produce C fibre firing. I have called this
pulvinar cell Type I as seen in Fig. 4. In addition to this, cells responsive
to sensory input in the pulvinar have been found that have a reciprocal
reaction to C fibre input, that is, the resting rate of firing is abolished
by C fibre input as seen in Fig. 5. The duration of inhibition of this
Type II cell is for approximately the same duration of time as the

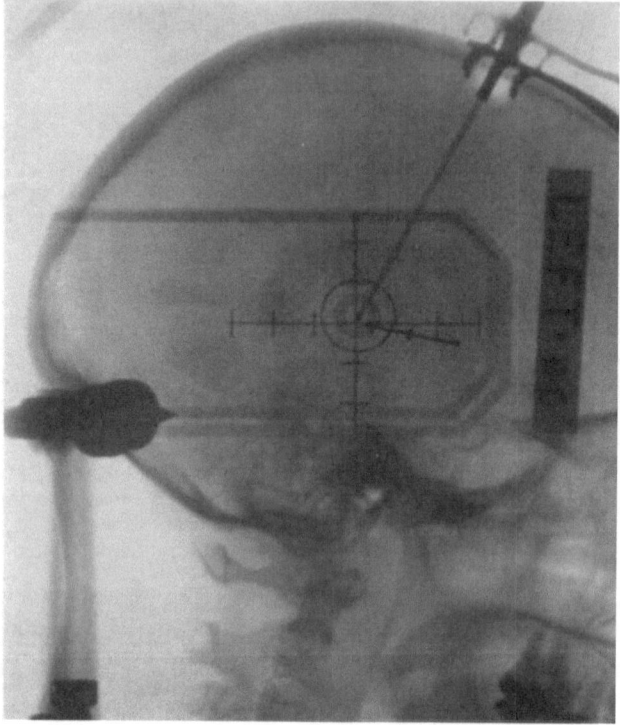

Fig. 6. Radiofrequency probe in anterior medial pulvinar (Fp = 15, Ht = 0)

activation of Type I cell, that is between 3 and 6 minutes. The implication of these two types of cells, of course, is that C fibre firing through
the reticular formation either inhibits the cell that ceases firing or
facilitates the cell that commences firing or both. Whether this is a
pathway to consciousness via the pulvinar to the parietal cortex,
frontal cortex, and limbic system is not known at this time. The pulvinar
may be acting as a facilitatory centre for the activation of other mechanisms for the perception of painful stimuli or for sustaining of systems
necessary for perception of pain.

At this time the primary drawback of operations on the sensory system at the level of the thalamus is that over prolonged period of time the chronic pain response begins to return. All patients operated either in the centre median, pulvinar, or a combination of both have had some return of pain over a 2–12 month period of time. In an attempt to prolong the period of pain relief, simultaneous lesions in the centre median and pulvinar have been used as well as bilateral lesions, both

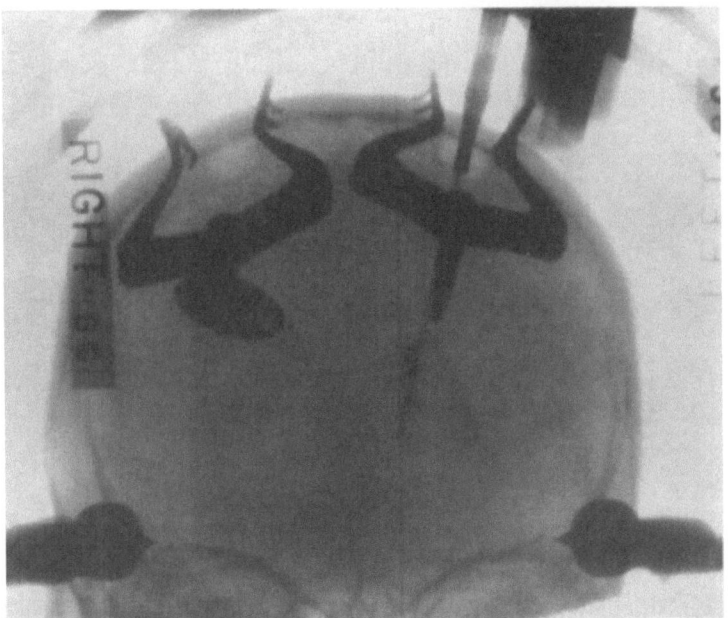

Fig. 7. Anterior view of probe in anterior medial pulvinar (Lat. = 12)

seem to have some additive effect, but the number of patients is too small for significant results at this time.

The implication of the return of pain is that either the projection of fibres carrying painful sensation is so diffuse through the thalamus that only a portion of the system is destroyed by lesions in the centre median and pulvinar which can later be circumvented by re-routing of impulses, or that lesions in these areas are not directly damaging the transmission pathways, but are systems necessary for gating of pain as Melzac and Wall[10] have found in the dorsal column of the spinal cord.

Discussion

The studies of Bishop[2], Bowsher[3, 4], Mehler[11], and Collins[5], have suggested that there are two pathways for painful sensation carried by the spinothalamic tract. Below the brain stem, anterolateral chordotomy relieves all types of pain with associated temperature loss demonstrating the unity of the two systems at this level. At the level of the brain stem, the more primitive system termed the paleospinothalamic pathway by Bishop[1] leaves the spinothalamic fibres and joins the reticular formation and should properly be termed the spinoreticular pathway. This multisynaptic unmyelinated path ascends to the centre median and pulvinar

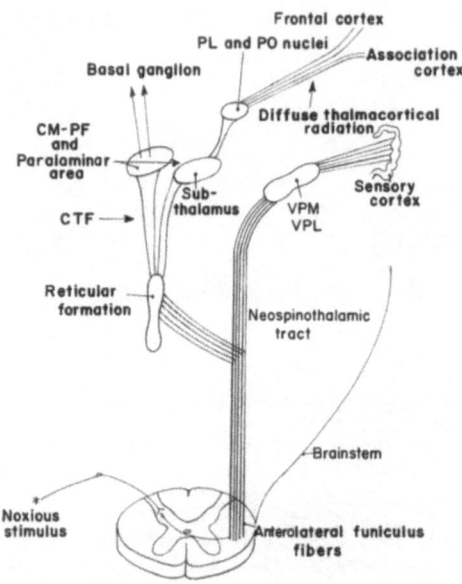

Fig. 8. Current concept of the central pathway for pain. The paliospinothalamic path is the contingent to the reticular formation and projection to the medial thalamus. *PL* pulvinar, *PO* posterior nuclear group, *CM-PF* centre median parafasicular complex (intralaminar nuclei), *CTF* central thalamic fasiculus, *VPM* ventral posterior medialis, *VPL* ventral posterior lateralis

of the thalamus where lesions produce loss of the slower, less well localized, protopathic pain typical of chronic pain of cancer with preservation of the epicritic pain sensation or lemniscal pathway to the ventral posterior nucleus of the thalamus which has been termed as the neospinothalamic system by Bishop[1].

Separation of the two pathways at the thalamic level allows destruction of at least a portion of the paleospinothalamic system with loss of chronic pain and preservation of all other sensation including epicritic pain, touch, proprioception, and temperature.

The stereotaxic procedure under local anesthesia is well tolerated by patients even with advanced cancer and carries a very low morbidity and mortality rate. Two patients have had thalamic haemorrhage following surgery with demise within hours following their surgery. The only other complication noted is that some patients have 2–3 days of mental confusion following their surgery, and two patients with hemiparesis. Patients with psychogenic pain neither have relief of their pain from thalamotomy from rhizotomy and chordotomy prior to attempted thalamotomy.

The single disadvantage of the procedure is the return of perception of chronic pain after several months which has kept thalamotomy from being a near ideal procedure for pain. Because of the return of pain it would be my recommendation that the procedure of sensory thalamotomy be reserved for patients with self-limiting illnesses such as recurrent cancer until more basic understanding of this system becomes available to allow permanent alleviation of pain by its manipulation. At present, unilateral or bilateral lesions combining destruction of the centre median and medial pulvinar seem to give the most complete and prolonged relief of pain, Fig. 6, 7, 8.

Summary

Stimulation and destruction of the intralamina area and medial pulvinar of the thalamus has proven these areas to be related to the perception of chronic pain. Relief of pain without detectable sensory loss can be obtained for several months with low morbidity. Basic studies in animals would indicate this pathway is from C fibre activation in the periphery and carried by the spinorecticular pathway through the ventral lateral columns of the spinal cord to the brain stem and upward through the reticular formation to the centre median, parafasicularis, and medial pulvinar of the thalamus. Above the thalamus, the pathway is poorly understood.

References

1. Bishop, G. H. (1959), The relationship between nerve fiber size and sensory modality: Phylogenetic implication of the afferent inervation of cortex. J. nerv. ment. Dis. *128*, 89—114.
2. — Landau, W. M. (1958), Evidence for a double peripheral pathway for pain. Science *128*, 712—713.
3. Bowsher, D. (1957), Termination of the central pain pathway in man: The conscious appreciation of pain. Brain *80*, 606—622.
4. — Petit, D., Malbart, G., Able-Fessard, D. (1968), A bulbar relay to the centre median. J. Neurophysiol. *31*, 288—300.
5. Collins, W. F., Nulsen, F. E. (1962), Studies on sensation interpreted pain: Central nervous system pathways. Clin. Neurosurg. *8*, 271—281.
6. — O'Leary, J. L. (1954), Study of a somatic evoked response in the midbrain reticular substance. EEG clin. Neurophysiol. *6*, 619—628.

7. Collins, W. F., Randt, C. T. (1958), Evoked central nervous system activity relating to peripheral unmyelinated or C fibers in cat. J. Neurophysiol. *21*, 345—352.
8. Landau, W., Bishop, G. H. (1953), Pain from dermal, periosteal and fascial endings and from inflammation. Arch. Neurol. Psychiat. *69*, 490—594.
9. Mark, V. H., Ervin, F. R., Yarkovlen, P. I. (1971), Correlation of pain relief, sensory loss, and anatomical lesion sites in pain patients treated by stereotaxic thalamotomy. Trans. Am. Neuro. Ass. *86*, 86—90.
10. Melzack, R., Wall, P. D. (1965), Pain mechanism: A new theory. Science *150*, 971—979.
11. Mehler, W. R. (1962), The anatomy of the so-called "pain tract" in man: An analysis of the course and distribution of the ascending fibers of fasiculus anterolateralis. Basic Research in Paraplegia, pp. 26—55. Charles C Thomas.
12. — Feferman, M. E., Nauta, W. J. H. (1960), Axon degeneration following anterolateral chordotomy in the monkey. Brain *83*, 718—750.
13. Petren, K. (1960), Über die Bahnung der Sensitivität im Rückenmark besonders nach dem Fallen von Strichverletzung studiert. Arch. Psychiat. *47*, 495.
14. Richardson, D. E. (1972), Sensory function of the pulvinar. Symposium on the Pulvinar St. Barnabar Hosp. N.Y., in press.
15. — (1972), Stereotaxic cingulumotomy and prefrontal lobotomy in mental disease. South. Med. J., in press.
16. — (1970), Sensory function of the pulvinar. Confin. Neurol. *32*, 165—173.
17. — (1967), Thalamotomy for intractable pain. Confin. Neurol. *29*, 139—145.

Author's address: D. E. Richardson, B.S., M.D., F.A.C.S. 1430 Tulane Avenue, New Orleans, LA 70112, U.S.A.

Acta Neurochirurgica, Suppl. 21, 89—91 (1974)
© by Springer-Verlag 1974

Department of Neurosurgery, University Central Hospital, Helsinki 26,
Finland

Combination of Thalamotomy and Longitudinal Myelotomy in the Treatment of Multiple Sclerosis

A Case Report

L. Laitinen, A. Arsalo, and A. Hänninen

Between 1964 and 1971, 30 patients with multiple sclerosis were referred to our neurosurgical department for the treatment of intention tremor, spasticity and intractable pain. Twenty-six patients underwent unilateral thalamotomy, 5 had longitudinal myelotomy of Bischof (Bischof, 1951; Laitinen and Singounas, 1971) and one had spinal commissurotomy. Two patients had both thalamotomy and longitudinal myelotomy.

The immediate clinical result was good in 73% of the 26 patients who were thalamotomized for intention tremor, *i.e.* the tremor of the contralateral arm was completely abolished. In 19% the result was fair, only slight tremor persisting, and in the remaining 8% the result of surgery was minimal. There was no surgical mortality. One patient had a postoperative extradural clot and 5 others showed some transitory hemiparesis. Two were confused and two showed dysphasia and dyspraxia, respectively.

At follow-up ranging from 8 months to 8 years, on the average 3.3 years, 7 patients had died from progression of the disease. Death had occurred 1 month to 7.5 years after surgery, on the average of 3.8 years. In 76% of the patients the tremor had remained absent. In 38% thalamotomy had caused permanent damage to speech (Arsalo et al., 1973).

All 5 patients who underwent longitudinal myelotomy of Bischof for severe spasticity of the legs had good immediate results; the spasticity was completely abolished. Although some recurrence of spasticity developed in the ankles during the follow-up period of 3–4 years, all patients were still pleased with the result of surgery. One patient who had thoracic commissurotomy for intractable pain of the pelvis had a slight recurrence after 2–3 months, but one year later he could still manage without analgesics.

Thalamotomy and longitudinal myelotomy were combined in two patients. In one of them the functional recovery was remarkably good and this case will be reported here:

Case Report

A. S., a woman of 28, had the first symptoms of M. S. when she was 19 years old. She suffered from rapidly progressing extension spasticity of the legs. Intention tremor appeared in the arms when she was 20. She soon became completely paraplegic and remained bedridden for 8 years. The intention tremor of the arms gradually increased and for 2 years she was unable to feed herself.

In June 1969 she was admitted to the Department of Neurosurgery in Helsinki. In both hands the intention tremor was so severe that she could not use her hands at all. The squeezing power of the hands was slightly weakened. Because of urinary incontinence she had an indwelling catheter in the bladder. Both legs were extremely spastic and hyperextended, and without any voluntary motility. The left leg ached. There was cutaneous sensory loss below the waist.

On 24 June 1969 left thalamotomy was carried out. The tremor of the right arm disappeared completely and she could start eating, writing and smoking.

Because the extension spasticity of the legs prevented her from sitting in a chair, dorsal longitudinal myelotomy, through D IX–XII laminectomy, was done on 23 October 1969. When she came round from the anaesthesia all spasticity was absent and next morning she could move her legs voluntarily. Six months later the muscle power of both legs had become almost normal and she could move freely in a wheel-chair. One year after surgery she could stand up and walk with a stick.

In August 1972, three years after surgery, we summoned the patient to the latest follow-up study. She arrived driving her own car. The motility of the legs was very good; only the sensory loss made the movements somewhat jerky and ataxic. Weak ankle reflexes were present, but no patellar reflexes. There was no tremor in the right arm, while the left was shaking. She still had an indwelling catheter in the bladder. Since January 1972 she had been working in an office of the University of Turku. She was a very happy woman, knitting even during the examination. She said that she was planning to get married.

Conclusions

Functional neurosurgery is relatively rarely indicated in the treatment of multiple sclerosis. The present study shows that thalamotomy may effectively and permanently abolish the intention tremor of one arm. The risks of thalamotomy are small. Longitudinal myelotomy may also permanently abolish the spasticity of the legs. In some cases, a

combination of these two operations may result in a remarkable restoration of functional health.

References

1. Arsalo, A., Hänninen, A., Laitinen, L. (1973), Functional neurosurgery
   in the treatment of multiple sclerosis. Ann. Clin. Res. *5,* 74—79.
2. Bischof, W. (1951), Die longitudinale Myelotomie. Zbl. Neurochir. *11,*
   79—88.
3. Laitinen, L., Singounas, E. (1971), Longitudinal myelotomy in the
   treatment of spasticity of the legs. J. Neurosurg. *35,* 536—540.

Authors' address: L. Laitinen, M.D., Department of Neurosurgery,
Topelius 5, Helsinki 26, Finland.

Acta Neurochirurgica, Suppl. 21, 93—100 (1974)

Neurosurgical University Clinic, Freiburg i. Br., Federal Republic of
Germany

Protracted Long-Term Irradiation
of Inoperable Midbrain Tumours
by Stereotactic Curie-Therapy using Iridium-192*

F. Mundinger and T. Hoefer

With 8 Figures

While the semimalignant gliomas of the diencephalon, mesencephalon
and cerebral trunk are inoperable by conventional neurosurgical methods,
resistant to treatment with external techniques of irradiation[2, 3, 4]
and can be freed of internal pressure only through fluid-drainage operations, they have long been the targets of stereotactic operational
treatment[13] principally using the method of implanting radioactive
gold-198 and yttrium-90 (Talairach and Szikla[14], Hankinson[1], and
others). We ourselves (Mundinger and Riechert) began using such
implantations in 1954[12]. Then starting in 1966 Mundinger undertook
to implant iridium-192, with its half-live of 74 days, into most of the
astroblastomas, oligoblastomas and spongioblastomas which we treated[10].
Prior to this we had gathered over 10 years of encouraging experience
with iridium-192, using it for irradiation of semimalignant trabecular
gliomas, gliomas of the hemisphere and pituitary adenomas[6, 7, 8, 9].
Since this form of protracted long-term irradiation[5] entails a relatively
slow dosage accumulation over a period of 7 months, there is a gradual
build-up of scar tissue and shrinkage of the tumour. Whereas the
short-lived radioisotopes mentioned have a necrotic effect, the iridium-192
irradiation causes devitalisation and thus protects to a great extent
the intact intermediate and surrounding neuronal structures and permits
compensating processes to develop. This explains why, clinically as well,
no reaction to irradiation is noted. The initially low sensitivity of these
tumour cells towards radioactivity increases as a result of the long-term

* Supported by a Special Research Programme ,,Gehirnforschung
und Sinnesphysiologie (SFB 70, III d)" of the Deutsche Forschungsgemeinschaft.

accumulation of irridiation doses, and thus they are more apt to be lethally affected by radioactivity than is the surrounding tissue. Moreover, continual emission of the doses ensures with great probability that the tumour cells in the periphery which have a premitotic pause will be lethally hit rather than the normal cells. This gives us an idea of the basically different radiobiologic mechanisms which are most advantageous for tumour localization. But it also makes it apparent that tumours showing malignant stigmata are unsuited for this type of long-term irradiation.

Three years ago in New York at the International Symposium for Stereoencephalotomy we made, together with Metzel, a first intermediate report on our results[11]. Since then we are in a position to survey our findings from 27 cases with postoperative observation times of up to 6 years and we may thus today make a more definite statement about the value of iridium-192 Curie-therapy in midline tumours.

R. B. Stereotactic Operation No. 39/67:

A space-occupying process located bilaterally in the thalamus of a 5-year-old girl in 1967 (Fig. 1). The little girl was marasmic and had to be fed artificially. She came to us with hemiparesis, athetotic hyperkinesia and a severe akinetic-mutistic psychoorganic syndrome. We made a stereotatic puncture into the centre of the tumour, taking minute biopsies along the length of the implantation. Histologic examination in squash-preparation revealed the presence of a spongioblastoma. An iridium-192 implantation was performed (Fig. 2). This and all other histologic examinations were performed for us by Prof. Noetzel and Doz. Dr. E. Metzel. The patient is now still alive 5 years subsequent to implantation and shows nearly complete involution of disruptive symptoms except for a remaining light paresis of the right nervus abducens. Two years ago we undertook to perform a re-implantation on account of the slow recurrent development of a psycho-organic syndrome. Since then the child has begun to develop again normally (Fig. 3). There is a whole series of similar examples.

Results

Localization and histology: In 15 out of 27 cases the tumour was localized in the region of the anterior third ventricle, principally in the hypothalamus but in 6 instances in the caudal thalamus and 6 further in the midbrain and rostral brain stem (Fig. 4).

Histologic examination revealed that the 6 astrocytomas and 6 spongioblastomas in the diencephalon were found 2–3 times more frequently than other types of tumour, for the most part oligodendrogliomas (Fig. 5). In the mesencephalon and cerebral trunk the difference in frequency was evidently less marked insofar as the limited number of cases permits us any judgment whatsoever.

Mortality: Three patients died in the hospital. One, suffering from a pineoblastoma and another one suffering from an astrocytoma, died

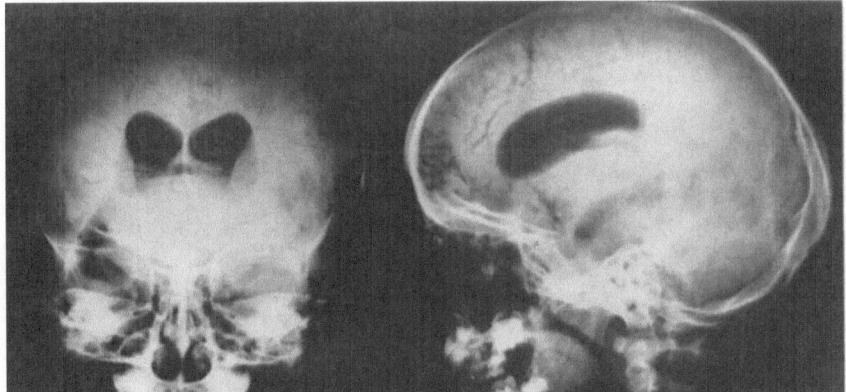

Fig. 1. B. R. 3 y. 6 m. (1967) Pneumoencephalography. Bilateral space-occupying process in the Thalamus

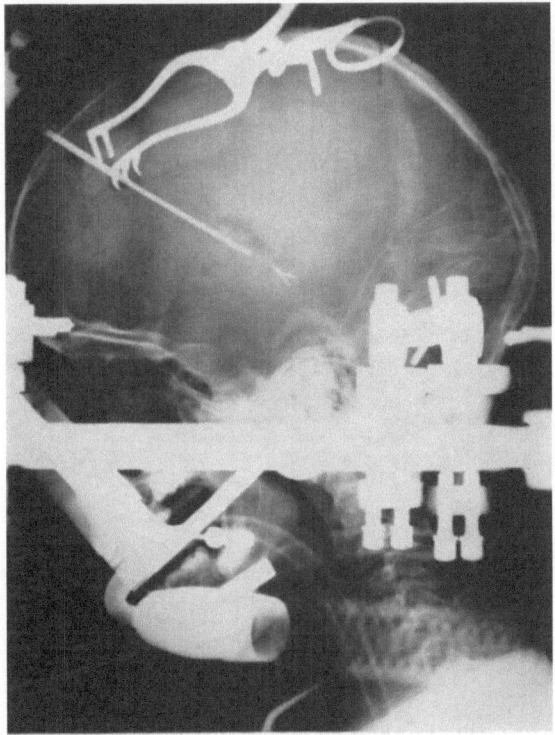

Fig. 2. B. R. 3 y. 6 m. X-ray photo with the implanted Ir-192 wires and sond

as the result of a haemorrhage followed by a ventricle tamponade probably due to the puncture or biopsy. The third one died following a later implantation of a atrio-ventricular shunt. In the period of 2 to

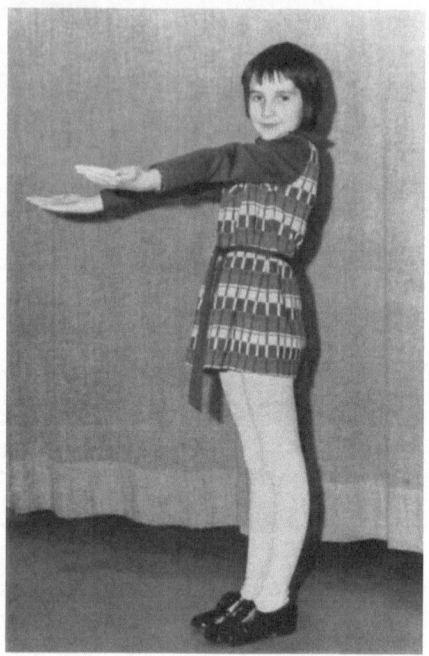

Fig. 3. B. R. Photo: 4 years and three months after first Ir-192-Implantation. Act. 4, 17 mCi (January 19th, 1967, Op. No. 39/67)

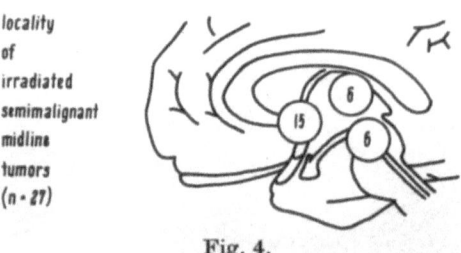

Fig. 4.

13 months after the implantation 6 patients died, 5 of whom were middle-aged or elderly. They had tumours mostly the size of a tangerine, and in two cases malignant, which *per se* no longer presents an indication for operation.

Survival times: As of July 31, 1972 the remaining 18 patients were still alive and their survival times ranged up to 72 months (Fig. 6).

For 13 patients, major symptoms such as seizures, visual disturbances, hyperkinesias, pareses, intracranial pressure and psycho-organic

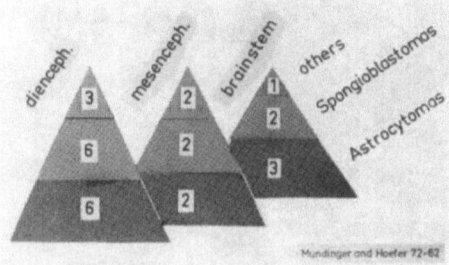

Fig. 5. Stereotactic Iridium-192 Curie-Therapy of inoperable semimalignant midline tumours (n = 27)

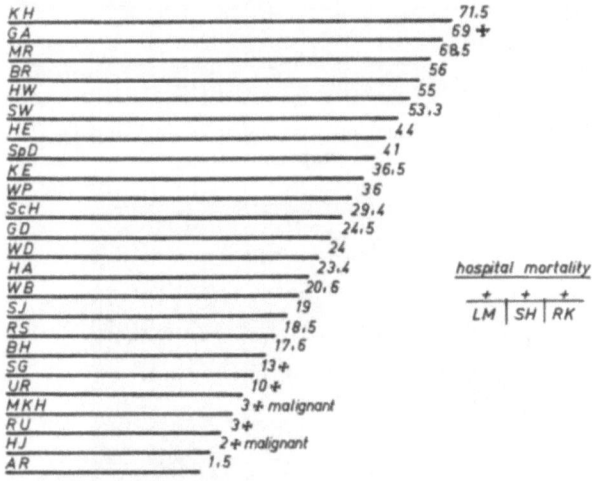

Fig. 6. Survival time of irradiated midbrain tumours (n = 27)

disturbances have greatly improved or subsided altogether (Fig. 7). For one patient, indicated here with a cross, the excellent improvement of his symptoms continued until shortly before his death 5 years later. Good improvement was registered for 3 patients and for 2 others temporarily prior to their deaths.

6 patients showed no improvement at all. In 5 of these our operation was preceded by an open operation which had led in part to a massive decline in symptoms. Thus the starting conditions for stereotactic

implantation were unfavourable, as a comparison with the other cases
shows.

This final diagram provides a survey of the results of treatment
(Fig. 8).

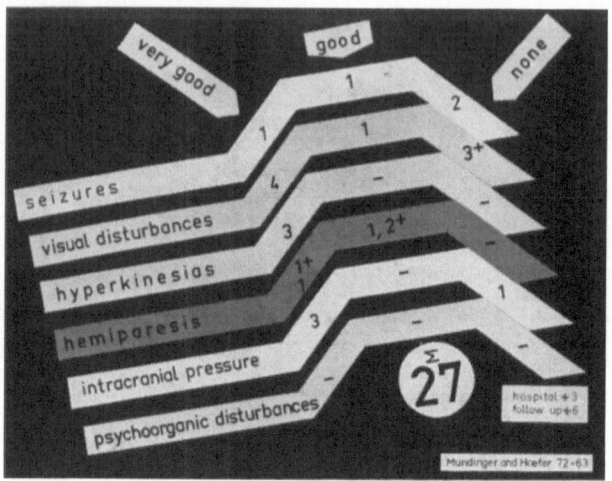

Fig. 7. Curie-Therapy effect on main neurological and psychoorganic
symptoms

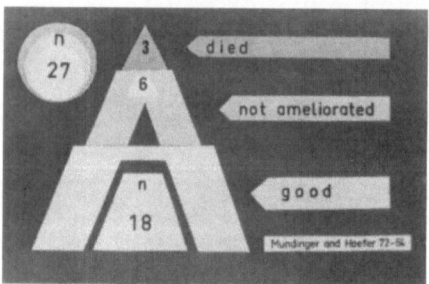

Fig. 8. Results of treated cases

At this point it might be argued that since these tumours grow very
slowly, cerebrospinal fluid-drainage might well have accomplished the
same involution of symptoms. This can certainly be said of the 3 cases
in which cerebral pressure had been clinically manifested as a result of
an otdurating hydrocephalus. But in only half of the cases, a total
of 12, did we perform an atrio-ventricular shunt. We laid the shunt
2 weeks to a maximum of 2 years prior to iridium-192 implantation
for 6 patients. 5 of the 6 subsequently regained better general health
and were free of complaints. However, the neurologic and psychic

symptoms of disruption continued to progress or remained unchanged. For the other 6 cases we installed the shunt prophylactically after the iridium implantation, having ascertained by direct measurement during the stereotactic operation higher pressure (CSF) in the ventricle. Consequently, we may affirm the necessity of including the drainage operation in the treatment plan, when such is called.

Local symptoms, caused by the invasion of the tumour into, for example, the region of the oculomotor-nuclei or of the reticular system, to name the most important, recede as a result of the irradiation which brings about local diminution of pressure. This effect is confirmed by the slow and gradual improvement of symptoms over a period of several months, occurring in more or less direct proportion to the dosage accumulation of iridium-192 in the tumour.

Summary

On the basis of long-term postoperative observation of up to 6 years in 27 biopsied cases it may be noted that stereotactic Curie-therapy with iridium-192 for protracted long-term irradiation presents an effective, clinically relevant and palliative method of treatment for supratentorial, semimalignant gliomas of the middle line, tumours which are otherwise inoperable and resistant to conventional irradiation techniques.

References

1. Hankinson, J. (1961), Therapeutic isotopes. Excerpta medica (Amsterdam) Int. Congr. Series 36. II. Int. Congr. Neurochir. Washington.
2. Lindgren, M. (1958), On tolerance of brain tissue and sensitivity of brain tumours to irradiation. Acta radiol. (Stockholm) Suppl. 170.
3. — (1965), Die Strahlenbehandlung der Hirntumoren. Dtsch. Röntgenkongr. 1964, Teil B. Strahlenbehandlung und -biologie, S. 220—230. München und Berlin: Urban und Schwarzenberg.
4. Löhr, H.-H., Vieten, H. (1967), Die Strahlenbehandlung raumbeengender intracranieller Prozesse. In: Handbuch der Neurochirurgie, Bd. IV, S. 421—566. Berlin-Heidelberg-New York: Springer.
5. Mundinger, F. (1958), Beitrag zur Dosimetrie und Applikation von Radio-Tantal (Ta^{182}) zur Langzeitbestrahlung von Hirngeschwülsten. Fortschr. Röntgenstr. 89, 86—91.
6. — (1966), Treatment of brain tumors with radioisotopes; in Krayenbühl, Maspes and Sweet: Progress of neurological surgery, Vol. 1, pp. 101—145. Basel/New York: Karger.
7. — (1969), Techniques and indications for the interstitial irradiation of brain and pituitary tumours with radionuclides. Kerntechnik, Isotopentechnik und Chemie 11, 333—345.
8. — (1969), Die intraselläre protrahierte Langzeitbestrahlung von Hypophysenadenomen mittels stereotaktischer Implantation von Iridium^{192}. Acta radiol. (Stockholm) 8, 55—62.

9. Mundinger, F. (1970), The treatment of brain tumors with interstitially applied radioactive isotopes. In: Yen Wang and Paoletti Monograph: Radionuclide Applications in Neurology and Neurosurgery, pp. 199—265. Springfield, Ill.: Ch. C Thomas.
10. — Metzel, E. (1968), Erfahrungen mit der lokalen Strahlenbehandlung inoperabler Zwischenhirn- und Basalganglientumoren mit der stereotaktischen Permanent-Implantation von Iridium[192]. Arch. Psychiat. Nervenkr. *212*, 70—90.
11. — — (1970), Interstitial radioisotope therapy of intractable diencephalic tumors by the stereotaxic permanent implantation of Iridium[192], Including Biotic Control. 4th Symp. Int. Soc. Res. Stereoencephalotomy, New York 1969. Confin. Neurol. *32*, 195—202.
12. — Riechert, T. (1967), Hypophysentumoren-Hypophysektomie. Stuttgart: Thieme.
13. Riechert, T., Mundinger, F. (1959), Stereotaktische Geräte. In Schaltenbrand und Bailey: Einführung in die stereotaktischen Operationen mit einem Atlas des menschlichen Gehirns. Stuttgart: Thieme.
14. Talairach, J., Bonis, A., Szikla, G., Schaub, G., Bancaud, J., Covello, L., Bordas-Ferrer, M. (1970), Stereotaxic implantation of radioactive isotopes in functional pituitary surgery: technique and results; in Yen Wang and Paoletti Monograph: Radionuclide Applications in Neurology and Neurosurgery, pp. 267—299. Springfield, Ill.: Ch. C Thomas.
15. Vieten, H., Löhr, H.-H. (1965), Probleme und Möglichkeiten der Strahlenbehandlung von Hirntumoren. Nervenarzt *36*, 429—437.

Authors' address: Prof. Dr. F. Mundinger and Dr. T. Hoefer, Neurosurgical Clinic, University of Freiburg, Hugstetterstraße 55, D-7800 Freiburg/Brsg., Federal Republic of Germany.

Acta Neurochirurgica, Suppl. 21, 101—110 (1974)

Department of Neurosurgery, Institute of Neurology, Queen Square,
London, England, and
The Regional Centre for Neurology and Neurosurgery, Oldchurch Hospital,
Romford, Essex, England

The Position and Extent of the Human Dentate Nucleus

P. Gortvai and S. Teruchkin

With 4 Figures

There have been several accounts in the literature in recent years of
the relief of spasticity and of movement disorders by surgical destruction
of all or part of the dentate nucleus (Toth 1961, Heimburger 1967,
Zervas et al. 1967, Siegfried et al. 1970). Thalamic lesions have been
known to alleviate rigidity and involuntary movement, but in most,
if not all cases, a thalamic lesion fails to improve spasticity and some
types of involuntary movement, especially choreoathetosis (Gortvai
1964). The failure of thalamotomy in such cases provides one of the
driving forces in the search for another neuronal system as the target
for therapeutic stereotactic surgery.

Previous work provides measurements and co-ordinates of the
dentate nucleus (Heimburger and Whitlock 1965, Slaughter and
Nashold 1968). We felt that before attempting stereotactic surgery,
we should ourselves attempt to measure the position and extent of the
dentate nucleus and form an idea of its variability.

The purpose of this communication is to summarize the results of
our measurements.

Material and Methods

Nine cerebellar hemispheres were examined in this study. Having
discarded specimens which were technically unsatisfactory, the right and
left sides were treated as equivalent. Table 1 shows data on age, sex and
side relating to the specimens.

The brains were removed from the corpses when the cause of death was
other than a neurological condition and were immersed in a solution of
8% formaldehyde in saline, with a phosphate buffer at pH 7 to which
saturated sodium chloride solution was added until the brain floated freely

P. Gortvai and S. Teruchkin:

Table 1. *Cerebellar Hemispheres Studied*

Specimen number	Age	Sex	Side
2	66	F	L
3	54	F	R
5	48	F	R
6	48	F	L
7	63	M	R
8	63	M	L
9	49	M	L
10	49	M	R
11	50	F	R

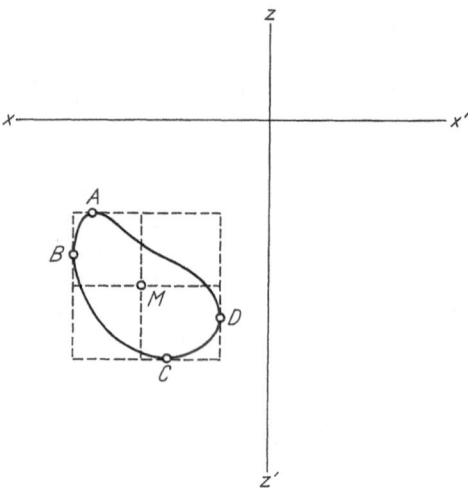

Fig. 1. Diagram of the dentate nucleus in the horizontal plane. $x - x^1$ is a line along the plane of the floor of the 4th ventricle, $z - z^1$ marks the midline. A, B, C and D are the outermost limits of the nucleus. M is the mid-point of the nucleus. These reference points were measured

without distortion. Within two weeks the brains were removed from the solution and sectioned. Immersion for such a comparatively short time does not fix the tissues but merely preserves them, and causes virtually no shrinkage. Shrinkage of brains immersed for such a short time was found to be less than 5%, mostly only 2% (Andrew and Watkins 1969) and we confirmed it by direct linear measurements.

The brains were cut at the level of the superior colliculi and the distal parts preserved. The cerebellum and brain-stem were bisected exactly down the midline at the sagittal plane. Specimens where the cut did not bisect the cerebral acqueduct and the 4th ventricle were discarded. Each suitable cerebellar hemisphere was then cut along the horizontal plane passing through the fastigium of the 4th ventricle exactly at right angles to the tangential plane of the floor of the 4th ventricle, with the aid of guide-lines on the cutting board and an open-ended box to define the desired plane. The cut surface was used as a reference plane and called P_0 plane subsequently. Blocks 3×2 cm in cross-section and 1.5 cm thick were cut—the superior block labelled A, the inferior block P. Each block was put in a freezing microtome and pared down at 20 micron intervals. The blocks were photographed each time after cutting away 0.1 cm. On these unstained surfaces the outline of the dentate nucleus was clearly visible and photographed well with flash equipment. Photographs were thus obtained of the cross-section of the nucleus at 0.1 cm intervals without tissue wastage. The photographs were enlarged at exactly $5 \times$ linear magnification, checked by incorporating a metric scale on the photographs.

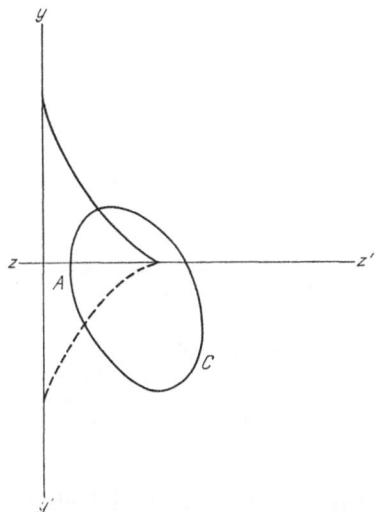

Fig. 2. Diagram of the dentate nucleus in the sagittal plane. $y — y^1$ runs along the floor of the 4th ventricle, $z — z^1$ through the fastigium of the 4th ventricle. A and C are the lateral limits of the nucleus

Translucent paper, lined at 0.1 cm intervals, was placed on each photograph in which the dentate nucleus appeared and the outlines of the nucleus were traced, together with the midline and the tangential line along the floor of the 4th ventricle.

The distance of the four outermost limits of the nucleus, like the four points of the compass, were measured from above reference lines.

The midpoint of the nucleus was calculated from these measurements as the point halfway between the outermost limits.

Fig. 1 shows the reference points measured and the derivation of the mid-point.

The area of each section was determined by counting the number of squares on the ruled-out tracing paper covering it.

Results

In the *sagittal plane* the lateral borders of the dentate nucleus were obtained by measuring points A and C from the vertical tangential line along the floor of the 4th ventricle ($y-y^1$). The relationship of these geometrical loci is illustrated in Fig. 2.

Graph 1 shows the mean measurements, with their standard deviations added as error-bars. The nucleus extends from 0.5 cm to 2.1 cm from the

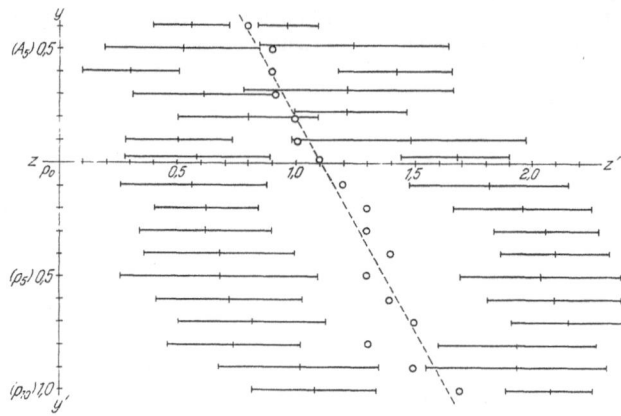

Graph 1. The borders of the dentate nucleus in the sagittal plane, orientated as in Fig. 2. The horizontal lines across the measurements of the borders represent twice the standard deviation. The open circles are the mean mid-points, and the interrupted line across them is the mean central axis

floor of the fourth ventricle. The standard deviations are of the order of 0.2 cm. The nucleus is oval in profile, and is inclined at an angle of 29° to the floor of the 4th ventricle. The mean mid-points of the nucleus, calculated according to Fig. 1, are also shown on the graph and a line across them gives the longitudinal axis of the nucleus. The axis is 29° to the floor of the fourth ventricle. The vertical extent of the nucleus is not taken into consideration. The error-bars separate between P_3 and P_6, 0.3 and 0.6 cm below the fastigial line, giving the best probability to enter the nucleus.

In the coronal plane the lateral borders of the nucleus are measured as points B and D from the midline ($y-y^1$). Fig. 3 illustrates the geometry.

The mean measurements are shown in Graph 2, with standard deviations as error-bars. The lateral borders of the nucleus extend from 0.5 cm to 2 cm from the midline, with a standard error of the order of 0.2 cm. The mean mid-points are also plotted at each level at 0.1 cm intervals, and the line across the mid-points, the longitudinal axis of the nucleus, forms an angle of 30 degrees with the midline. As in the sagittal plane, the error-bars separate between P_3 and P_6, that is 0.3 and 0.6 cm below the fastigial line.

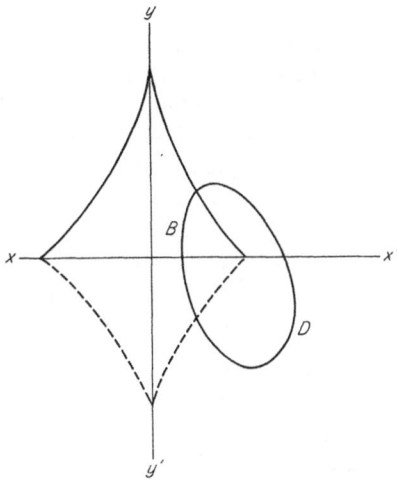

Fig. 3. Diagram of the dentate nucleus in the coronal plane. $y - y^1$ is the midline, $x - x^1$ the line through the fastigium of the 4th ventricle. B and D are the lateral borders of the nucleus

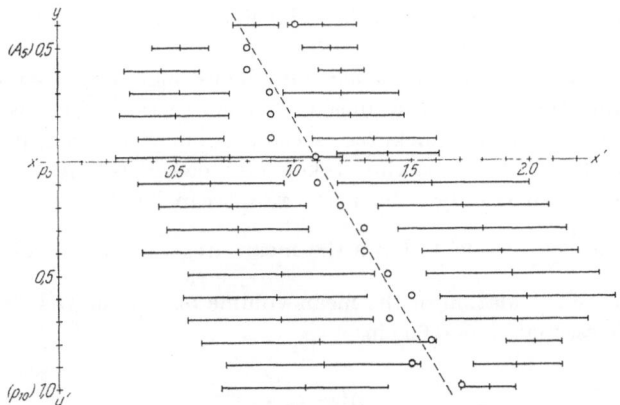

Graph 2. The borders of the dentate nucleus in the coronal plane, orientated as in Fig. 3. The horizontal lines across the measurements of the borders represent twice the standard deviation. The open circles are the mean midpoints, and the interrupted line across them is the mean central axis

P. Gortvai and S. Teruchkin:

The mean mid-points of the nucleus are presented in Table 3.

The mean *longitudinal extent* of the nucleus is 1.2 cm, but it varies from 0.9 to 1.6 cm, the cranial end from 0 to 0.6 cm above the fastigal plane, and the caudal end 0.6 to 1.0 cm below that plane. The measurements relating to individual specimens are given in Table 2. There is more variation along the longitudinal axis than in the lateral directions.

Table 2. *Showing the Longitudinal Extent and Position of the Dentate Nucleus.* The Mean midpoint is at P_3 (3 mm below the Plane Passing through the Fastigium)

Brain	Cranial (A)	Mid-point	Caudal (P)	Total length
3	6	p^2	10	16
2	6	p^0	6	12
6	3	p^4	10	13
5	3	p^3	9	12
7	5	p^0	5	10
9	2	p^3	7	9
10	0	p^5	10	10
8	3	p^4	10	13
11	3	p^4	10	13
Mean	3.4	P^3	8.6	12

The mean mid-point along this axis is at P_3, 0.3 cm below the fastigial line, but P_5, 0.5 cm below the fastigial line is also shared by all speciments.

The mean *volume* of the nucleus may be estimated approximately by determining the area of the nucleus at each section, then multiplying by 0.1 cm, that is the thickness of the section. The maximum extent of the nucleus, 1.6 cm, is thus taken into consideration, but because the mean length is only 1.2 cm, the result can be corrected by multiplying with $\frac{1.2}{1.6}$. Table 4 shows the mean areas at each level, and the approximate calculation of the mean volume of the nucleus. The mean volume is estimated as 0.66 cm³.

Discussion

The geometrical mid-point of the dentate nucleus can be plotted in the coronal plane and the sagittal plane with the lateral borders having only a standard deviation of 0.2 cm. Along the vertical axis the nucleus

Table 3. *Showing the Mean Mid-point of the Dentate Nucleus from the Midline (along $x - x^1$ Axis) and from the Floor of the 4th Ventricle (along $z - z^1$ Axis), in cms*

	A6	A5	A4	A3	A2	A1	P0	P1	P2	P3	P4	P5	P6	P7	P8	P9	P10
From midline	1.0	0.8	0.9	0.9	0.9	0.9	1.1	1.1	1.2	1.3	1.3	1.4	1.5	1.4	1.6	1.5	1.4
From floor of 4th ventricle	0.8	0.9	0.9	0.9	1.0	1.0	1.1	1.2	1.3	1.3	1.4	1.3	1.4	1.5	1.3	1.5	1.7

Table 4. *Showing the Mean Areas of the Dentate Nucleus in Horizontal Sections, and a Calculation to Arrive at an Approximate Volume*

	A6	A5	A4	A3	A2	A1	P0	P1	P2	P3	P4	P5	P6	P7	P8	P9	P10
Mean area of cross-section in cm²	0.25	0.30	0.36	0.36	0.36	0.43	0.46	0.53	0.65	0.61	0.80	0.72	0.76	0.60	0.66	0.60	0.40

Volume = sums of mean areas $\times$ 0.1 cm = 0.88 cm³, but mean length is 1.2 cm, not 1.6 cm, therefore: volume = $0.83 \times \dfrac{1.2}{1.6}$ cm³ = 0.66 cm³.

is more variable. The figures of Heimburger and Whitlock (1965) refer to a vertical plane which passes through the fastigium.

Slaughter and Nashold (1968) use the tangenital line of the 4th ventricle as the vertical reference line, and in this study their reference here is retained. We felt that the floor of the 4th ventricle is more likely to be demonstrable with certainty on a radiological study, also we felt that it is likely to be less variable than the fastigium as a vertical reference plane.

Our co-ordinates differ somewhat from Slaughter and Nashold (1968). The central axis in our measurements subtends an angle less than theirs in both coronal and sagittal planes. Since the best chance of stereotactic surgery lies in attempting to introduce the electric probe along the central axis, the angle is of some importance. It is possible that the difference is introduced by the method used. We believe our method to be reasonably accurate, although necessarily open to criticism.

The midpoint of the dentate nucleus lies 0.3 cm below the fastigial line in our study. We believe that if a single aiming point is sought, 0.5 cm below the fastigial lines presents a better aiming co-ordinate, because here the certainty of being in the nucleus is greater, also using 0.5 cm below the fastigial line increases the distance from the mid-line, thus getting the operator further away from the small cerebellar nuclei because of the angle of the central axis of the nucleus with the midline and the floor of the 4th ventricle. At 0.5 cm below the fastigial plane the mid-point of the nucleus lies at 1.4 cm posterior to the floor of the 4th ventricle and 1.4 cm from the midline, expressed as the mean.

The variability of the position of the nucleus along the vertical axis might explain the differing clinical results obtained by different investigators. Fortunately post-mortem material after operation is rare—but Heimburger and Whitlock (1965) describe a single case in which a postortem examination was obtained. On one side one-third of the nucleus was destroyed at surgery, on the other side the lesion missed the nucleus.

Physiological observations during stereotactic surgery could, we hope, usefully assist the anatomical findings in clinical cases. Some physiological results are given by Siegfried et al. (1970), such as stimulation and recording of electrical impulses.

Summary

A method is described briefly to prepare specially orientated photographs to determine the position and extent of the human dentate nucleus.

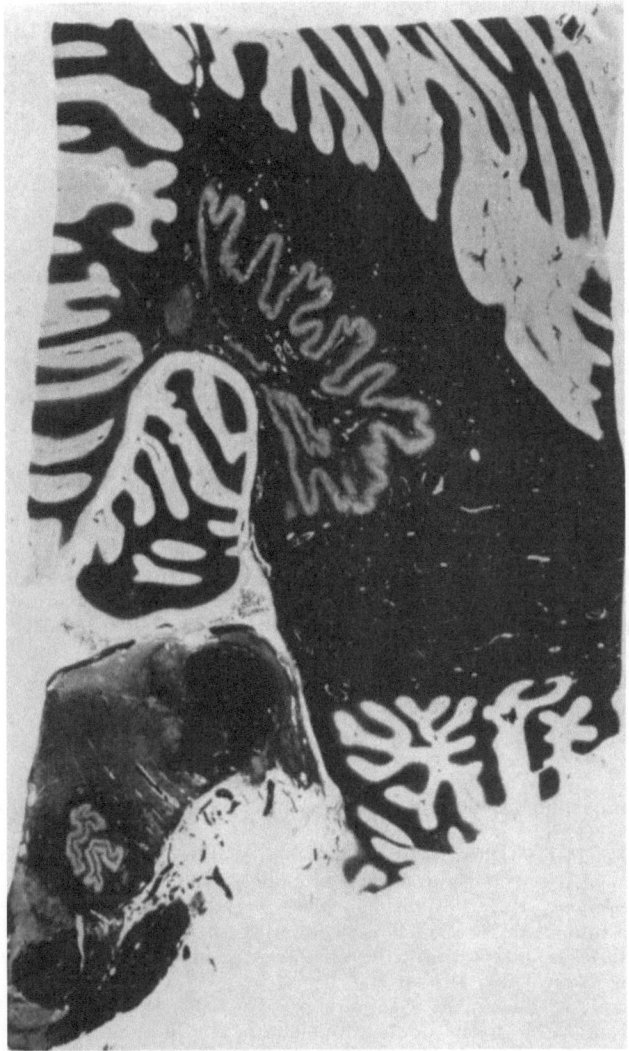

Fig. 4. Section of the cerebellum and brainstem in the horizontal plane through a block cut according to the method described. The section is taken 0.5 cm below the fastigial line. It is stained by the Loyez method, but measurements were made on frozen unstained material

The following main conclusions are made:

1. The dentate nuclei are oval structures, on each side of the 4th ventricle.

2. The lateral limits of the nuclei extend from 0.5 cm to 2.0 cm from the midline in the coronal plane, 0.5 cm to 2.1 cm from the floor of the 4th ventricle in the sagittal plane.

3. The standard deviation of lateral borders is of the order of 0.2 cm.

4. The longitudinal extent is variable from 0 to 0.6 cm above fastigial line and 0.5 to 1.0 cm below fastigial line. The mean length is 1.2 cm.

5. The longitudinal axis lies at 29° with floor of 4th ventricle and 30° with midline.

6. The geometrical centre is 0.3 cm below the fastigial line, 1.2 cm posterior to the floor of 4th ventricle and 1.2 cm from midline.

7. For a single aiming point 0.5 cm below fastigial line, 1.4 cm posterior to the floor of 4th ventricle and 1.4 cm from the midline may be preferable.

8. The approximate mean volume of the nucleus is 0.66 cm³.

Acknowledgement

We are grateful to the Institute of Neurology, Queen Square, and Professor Valentine Logue, for support and facilities, aided by a grant from the Department of Health and Social Security for locally organised research, and to the Department of Pathology, Oldchurch Hospital, Romford Essex for supplying the specimens and allowing us to use their facilities.

References

1. Andrew, J., Watkins, E. S. (1969), A stereotaxic atlas of the human thalamus and adjacent structures, p. 3. Baltimore: The Williams and Wilkins Co.
2. Gortvai, P. (1964), Surgery in disorders of movement other than Parkinsonism. J. Neurol. Neurosurg. Psychiat. *27*, 585—586.
3. Heimburger, R. F., Whitlock, C. C. (1965), Stereotaxic destruction of the human dentate nucleus. Confin. Neurol. *26*, 346—358.
4. — (1967), Dentatectomy in the treatment of dyskinetic disorders. Confin. Neurol. *29*, 101—106.
5. Siegfried, J., Esslen, E., Gretener, V., Ketz, E., Perret, E. (1970), Functional anatomy of the dentate nucleus in the light of stereotaxic operations. Confin. Neurol. *32*, 1—10.
6. Slaughter, D. G., Nashold, Jr. B. S. (1968), Stereotactic co-ordinates for the human dentate nucleus. Confin. Neurol. *30*, 375—384.
7. Toth, S. (1961), The effect of the removal of the nucleus dentatus on the parkinsonian syndrome. J. Neurol. Neurosurg. Psychiat. *24*, 143—147.

Authors' address: P. Gortvai, M.D., M. Chir., F.R.C.S., Regional Centre for Neurology and Neurosurgery, Oldchurch Hospital, Romford, Essex, England.

Acta Neurochirurgica, Suppl. 21, 111—117 (1974)
© by Springer-Verlag 1974

Departments of Surgery, Physiology, and Electrical Engineering,
University of Toronto, and Neurosurgical Unit, Toronto General Hospital,
Toronto, Canada

Physiological Guidelines for the Localization of Lesions by Percutaneous Cordotomy

R. R. Tasker, L. W. Organ, and K. C. Smith

With 1 Figure

Spinothalamic tractotomy, theorectically, is an ideal operation for the relief of intractable pain. But not until the introduction of the percutaneous technique by Mullan et al. (1963) could its benefits be extended to the majority of cancer patients; for most of them are too ill for open surgery. Moreover the precision of the new technique increases its effectiveness and at the same time minimizes complications.

After preliminary experience with 29 percutaneous cordotomies, we adopted the lateral C 1 C 2 approach and the protocol for electrode localization outlined by Taren et al. (1969) using biplanar X-rays, electrical impedance and spinal cord stimulation. 140 additional procedures have been done by these means, 90% for pain due to carcinoma, more than half lesions of cervix or rectum.

This account summarizes the results and then retrospectively examines the role of stimulation, the single most valuable tool, in the identification of the lateral spinothalamic fibres and the avoidance of the corticospinal tract.

Method

Percutaneous cordotomy is performed under fentanyl neuroleptanalgesia with local infiltration of 2% lidocaine hydrochloride and norepinephrine. Prior sedation is avoided. Image intensification in the lateral projection guides the introduction of a sharp, thin-walled, 18 lumbar puncture needle into the mid-anteroposterior plane of the appropriate C 1 C 2 interspace. The needle is supported on an upright post capable of fine three-dimensional manipulation. As soon as the subarachnoid space is entered, sufficient myelodil*, shaken up with a little normal saline solution and air, is injected to outline the dura, spinal cord, and, hopefully, dentate ligament. Previous horizontal alignment of the upper cervical spine facilitates the contrast study. The horizontal progression of the needle is followed with spot, rapid-process, antero-posterior, X-ray films; cord contact takes place when the needle tip lies about the centre of the image of the odontoid process. Upon completion of the myelography, the stilette of the L. P. needle is replaced by the cordotomy electrode, an electrolytically sharpened 0.4 mm stainless steel wire projecting 2 mm beyond the tip of its tubular teflon insulation. The insulation in turn projects 2 mm beyond the tip of the L. P. needle as shown in Fig. 1. Electrical impedance is continously monitored as the whole assembly is advanced under image intensification to just anterior to the dentate ligament. If the latter has not been outlined its position must be estimated. Impalement of the cord is usually palpable as the impedance rises, at first slowly, and then rapidly, from the 400 w characteristic of CSF to the 1200–1400 w of cord. The collar effect of the teflon tubing arrests the progress of the electrode so that its tip always comes to lie suspended 2 mm deep to the pia. Care is taken to avoid further penetration, for effective destruction of any part of the spinothalamic tract can be achieved at this depth and elimination of one dimension of electrode movement simplifies localization. Trains of 3 msec negative rectangular waves, first at 2 then at 100 Hz are used for stimulation while voltage is gradually increased to threshold or to about 4 volts**. Motor effects are observed while the patient is questioned about any sensory experience. Both motor and sensory effects are nearly always seen. Radiofrequency lesions are made at 30 mA for 30 seconds while the patient's ipsilateral motor power is monitored. Local neck pain and discomfort in the contralateral half of the body which may accompany lesion-making are best anticipated with additional injections of fentanyl. The patient is examined to ensure that analgesia to superficial and deep pain and to heat has been produced in the desired dermatomes and the lesion is increased, usually after repositioning the electrode, only if the initial effect is inadequate. It is seldom possible to enlarge the lesion by raising the current above 30 mA. Impedance, stimulation, and lesion-making are provided by a commercially available instrument***. If bilateral pain requires repetition of the procedure on the second side, this is done after a week's interval exactly as before,

---

* Glaxo-Allenbury brand of iophendylate.

** With our equipment 1 volt results in approximately 1 mA current flow.

*** The Owl Cordotomy System, 4634 Yonge Street, Willowdale, Ontario, Canada.

except that the patient is carefully monitored for 3–5 days post-opera-tively for evidence of inadequate ventilation. A rare complication, we feel that its risk after bilateral procedures is more than compensated for by the unique degree of precision afforded by the lateral C 1 C 2 approach.

Fig. 1. The cordotomy electrode (above) showing the 2 mm projection of its sharpened tip beyond its tubular insulation which in turn projects 2 mm beyond the tip of the L.P. needle when the electrode is inserted into the latter in place of the stilette

Results

A total of 78 consecutive procedures, 23 on the second side of the body, was attempted up until January 1, 1972 using the above method. The spinothalamic tract was identified at operation in 96%, two of the three failures occurring in confused unco-operative patients. At the time of discharge 93% of operations had resulted in the relief of the pain for which they had been performed, and at latest follow-up, 84% were still successful. Though occasionally pain relief was achieved with lesser degrees of sensory loss, it was most certain when sufficient analgesia had been produced in the painful dermatomes so that skin perforation with a hat pin and maximal manual compression of achilles tendon, a digit, or of subcutaneous tissue was not painful and radiant heat could not be identified until sufficient to cause discomfort in normal skin. Pain persistance was associated with less than this degree of analgesia in 80% of cases. Adequate analgesia was readily achieved from C6 derma-tome distally, with less certainty in C5, and only occasionally in C4. There was a slightly greater incidence of failure in lumbosacral than in cervicothoracic dermatomes.

Complications were few even though 20% of the operations were performed on bedridden patients, and most were able to return home post-operatively. There was one death arising from reduced ventilation, one case of reversible hypoventilation, one of reversible acute hydro-cephalus presumably due to haematoma of the cisterna magna. Four per cent of procedures resulted in loss of bladder control, all but 1 after lesions on the second side. The risk was greatest when there were pre-existing disturbances of micturition. Transient paresis was seen after 6% of operations but not a single case of persistent significant weakness. Post-cordotomy dysaesthesia occurred after 10% and was a significant disability after 3%; 21% resulted in Horner's syndrome.

Stimulation: During the first consecutive 100 cases, the cord was stimulated at 365 sites, and a lesion was made at 162. An attempt was made to localize all sites as anterior to, posterior to, or within the lateral spinothalamic tract on the basis of analgesia produced if a lesion had been made at that site, or by reference to another site at which a lesion had produced analgesia. 146 sites with lesions and 127 without could be so characterized.

Motor effects were studied first, 95% being ipsilateral. At 2 Hz the threshold required to produce a motor response was lower (less than 1 mA in half) for points anterior to spinothalamic tract than for those within or posterior to tract. The pattern of motor response was also helpful. Within or anterior to tract, 75% of motor responses with 2 Hz stimulation were confined to cervical muscles, especially trapezius, the rest involving usually in addition, hand or upper limb. Virtually none involved trunk or lower limb. At posterior sites however, 1/3 of the responses involved trunk or lower extremity. Surprisingly, when the stimulus frequency was increased to 100 Hz, motor responses (tetanization) were uncommon and precluded a satisfactory position when they did occur. Tetanization was seen at 24% of sites anterior to tract where neck muscles were involved, and 28% of sites posterior to tract when limbs or trunk were involved.

We concluded then that neck muscle contractions can occur above 1 mA with 2 Hz stimulation without tetanization with 100 Hz when the electrode lies in spinothalamic tract and must be due to stimulation of ventral horn or root by volume conduction. If the threshold is lower and/or tetanization of neck muscles occurs, the electrode lies anterior to tract where ventral horn or root are stimulated directly. Contractions of muscles in trunk or lower extremity with 2 Hz stimulation, usually accompanied by tetanization with 100 Hz stimulation, are seen when the electrode lies posteriorly and corticospinal tract is stimulated directly.

There is no obvious explanation for the contractions seen in the upper extremity with 2 Hz stimulation when the electrode lies in the spino-thalamic tract. More distal musculature is never involved and no tetanization is seen. Since these contractions often occur in myotomes as remote as those of the thenar muscles, stimulation of ventral horn or roots seem unlikely.

Whenever a lesion did produce paresis the latter was virtually restricted to the lower extremity and any associated analgesia occurred distally in the body. These observations are in keeping with the teaching that the most caudal fibres of the corticospinal and spinothalamic tracts abut at the level of the dentate ligament.

Sensory effects were examined next. Although sensory effects were produced by 2 Hz stimulation at 31% of sites within the spinothalamic tract, it was usually necessary to increase the rate of stimulation before a sensory experience was reported. We have arbitrarily used 100 Hz. Sensory threshold with 100 Hz stimulation was independent of the site stimulated, being less than 3 mA at 94% of them and usually less than 1 mA. Absence of a sensory response up to 4 mA as found at 5% of sites, precluded suitable positioning.

Strictly *ipsilateral* sensory responses were seen in sites posterior to spinothalamic tract, suggesting subthreshold stimulation of the corticospinal tract, an effect repeatedly observed with stimulation of the internal capsule during stereotactic surgery. Similar ipsilateral responses were also seen at anterior sites where they are more difficult to explain. Ipsilateral responses also occurred at 12% of sites within the spinothalamic tract but then always in association with more prominent contralateral responses. These could well be due to stimulation of ipsilateral spinothalamic fibres. Such a conclusion would be in keeping with identification of ipsilateral fibres in the spinothalamic tract in the midbrain and in the more posterior of the two somatotopographic representations of the body demonstrated in the human somatosensory thalamus[3, 4, 5, 6]. Stimulation of dorsal columns must be a rare occurrence but could account for some ipsilateral responses at posterior sites.

Once a contralateral sensory response had been obtained, careful questioning of the patient revealed that at 84% of sites in the spinothalamic tract, the experience was a sense of tingling associated with warmth or burning occasionally cold and pain. Usually only tingling, vibration, or mild electric shock were felt with stimulation elsewhere. Again, these observations parallel those made during stereotactic surgery in the midbrain and thalamus where stimulation of medial lemniscus and most of the somatosensory thalamus are reported as paraesthesia, and burning or temperature effects are restricted to spinothalamic tract and some thalamic points.

The location of the contralateral sensory effect was instructive. In half the sites anterior to tract, it was confined to the neck, but at only 2% of sites within the spinothalamic tract, and infrequently more posteriorly. Thus such a response indicates that the electrode lies too anteriorly. The physiological explanation for it is unclear, as it is for the bizarre sensory experiences often referred to the midline of the body seen in this same region.

8*

Contralateral sensory responses located more distally in the body virtually always occurred at sites within the spinothalamic tract, though rarely, presumably because of technical problems, a lesion made at an apparently ideal site might fail to produce analgesia. Surprisingly, the distribution of such stimulation-induced sensory effects did not necessarily conform to that of the analgesia produced by a lesion at the same site. However, an existing "level" of analgesia could be "raised" by extending the lesion that produced it anteriorly, or "lowered" by extending it posteriorly. Moreover, all dermatomal levels from C5 to sacral were accessible for lesion-making with the electrode tip 2 mm deep to pia. These findings suggest that the spinothalamic tract extends in a somatotopographically organized band of uniform depth in the antero-lateral quadrant of the cord.

When the sensory effect produced by stimulation was felt in the contralateral upper extremity, particularly the hand, a lesion at that site usually induced analgesia over most of the contralateral half of the body below C4. Half the sites where lesions produced such extensive analgesia were associated with stimulus-induced sensory responses in the upper limb compared with a quarter of the sites where lesions resulted in less complete analgesia. When the stimulus-induced contralateral sensory effect occurred distal to upper extremity, the lesion made at the same site was much more likely to induce analgesia more distally in the body, and most instances of leg paresis were associated with such sensory responses. From these observations we can conclude that direct stimulation of the spinothalamic tract usually gives rise to the contralateral experience of tingling and warmth or burning, the location of which is not necessarily the same as that of the analgesia produced by a lesion at the same site. Nevertheless, there is obvious anteroposterior somatotopy in the tract, most of which is occupied by fibres from the hand. Fibres from neck, trunk and lower limb occupy thin bands anterior or posterior as the case may be, to these central hand fibres a finding again reminiscent of the pattern seen in thalamus and midbrain. Thus, a 2–3 mm lesion centred in the hand fibres usually involves the more rostral and caudal fibres of the tract as well.

Summary

For practical purposes, with our equipment and technique, ideal location of the electrode in the central spinothalamic tract can be anticipated if the following observations are made with stimulation:

AT 2 HZ.

1. Contraction of ipsilateral neck muscles.
2. Especially trapezius.

3. At thresholds between 2–3 mA.

4. Simultaneous contralateral sensory experience is favourable.

At 100 HZ.

1. No tetanization.

2. A contralateral sensory experience.

3. Extending distal to neck.

4. Particularly in the hand.

5. At a threshold below 1 mA.

6. Described as tingling and warmth or burning.

Lesion-making should be avoided if:

1. Tetanization occurs at 100 Hz.

2. 2 Hz stimulation causes contractions in trunk or lower extremity.

3. In the absence of contralateral sensory effects below the neck at 100 Hz.

4. With extensive ipsilateral sensory effects.

References

1. Mullan, S., Harper, D. V., Hetmatpanah, J., Torres, H., Dobben, G. (1963), Percutaneous interruption of the spinal pain tracts by means of a strontium—90 needle. J. Neurosurg. *20*, 931—939.
2. Taren, J. A., Davis, R., Crosby, E. C. (1969), Target physiologic correlation in stereotaxic cervical cordotomy. J. Neurosurg. *30*, 569—584.
3. Tasker, R. R., Emmers, R. (1967), Patterns of somesthetic projection in SI and SII of the Human Thalamus. Confin. Neurol. *29*, 160 (abst.).
4. — — (1969), A double somatotopic representation in the human thalamus. Its application in localization during thalamotomy for Parkinson's disease. Proc. III. Symposium on Parkinson's Disease. Ed. J. Gillingham and M. L. Donaldson, 94—100. Edinburgh: E. and S. Livingstone Ltd.
5. — Richardson, P., Rewcastle, B., Emmers, R. (1972), Anatomical correlation of detailed thalamic sensory mapping in man. Confin. Neurol. *34*, 184—196.
6. — (1972), Mapping of the somatosensory and auditory pathways in the upper midbrain and thalamus in man. Neurophysiology studied in Man. Ed. Somjen, 169—187. Amsterdam: Excerpta Medica.

Authors' address: R. R. Tasker, M.D., Room 121 U.W., Toronto General Hospital, Toronto, Canada.

Acta Neurochirurgica, Suppl. 21, 119—123 (1974)
© by Springer-Verlag 1974

Department of Surgical Neurology, Western General Hospital, Crewe Road,
Edinburgh, Scotland

Physiological Correlates in Stereotactic Spinal Surgery

E. R. Hitchcock and Y. Tsukamoto

With 4 Figures

Stereotactic spinal surgery is a new and exciting field although it has still many problems to conquer. The main disadvantages which make some neurosurgeons prefer open cordotomy to the stereotactic procedure are the instability of the cord with penetration of the electrode and the comparatively small size of the target surrounded by other important pathways often with anatomical variations[5].

However this stereotactic procedure has definite advantages compared to open cordotomies since operation can be performed under local anaesthesia and the effects of stimulation and fractional lesion confirmed by questioning the patient. An additional advantage is that for patients with malignancy and in poor general condition the stereotactic procedure is less traumatic than the open.

More than 60 stereotactic cordotomies, spinothalamic tractotomy, commissural myelotomy[1, 3] and trigeminal tractotomy[2] have been performed since 1968 and these cases are reviewed chiefly in respect of physiological responses during stimulation of the cord. All procedures were performed using a specially designed spinal stereotactic instrument (Fig. 1).

There are two components in the instability of the cord during electrode penetration, displacement and rotation, which are accentuated in the extended position[3]. Taren[5] reported that electrodes push the cord more than 5 mm during the penetration of the pia mater. To lessen displacement therefore the patient's neck is flexed as much as possible and the needle inserted through the occipito-atlanto space. At this level and in the flexed position the medulla and the first segments of the cord are held relatively immobile by lower cranial nerves and by the large first dentate ligament. The electrode is insulated 0.5 mm diameter Tungsten with electrolytically sharpened tip of 10–50 μ.

E. R. Hitchcock and Y. Tsukamoto:

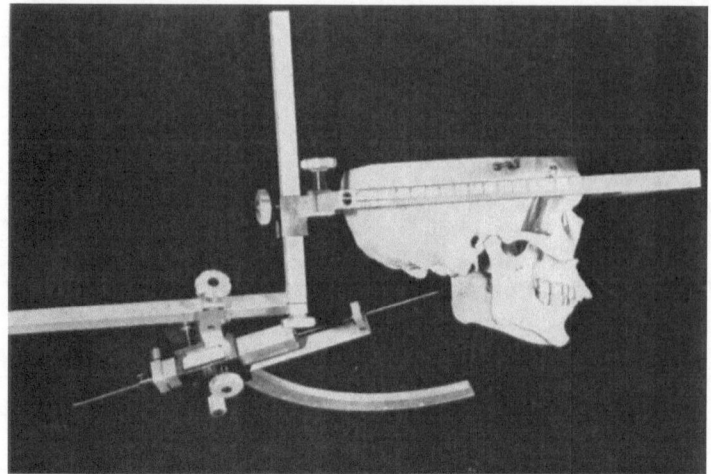

Fig. 1

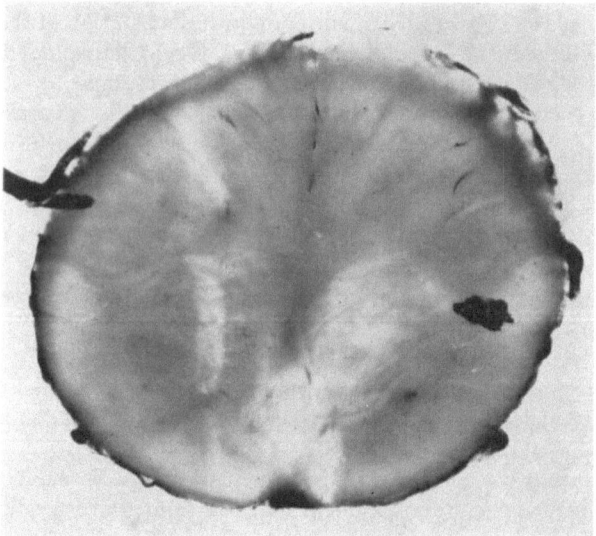

Fig. 2

Rotation of the cord is more difficult to control. Fig. 2 illustrates a post mortem confirmation of a central electrode track which is markedly curved due to rotation.

Naturally the degree of rotation is increased according to the increase of the "moment" around the centre of the cord (Fig. 3). Accordingly there is less rotation the nearer the electrode penetration is to the axis. The postero-anterior route therefore is preferred for commissuro-myelotomy, trigeminal tractotomy and spinothalamic tractotomy for the upper limbs and the lateral track for spinothalamic tractotomy of the lumbosacral pathway. Even using these procedures movement of the

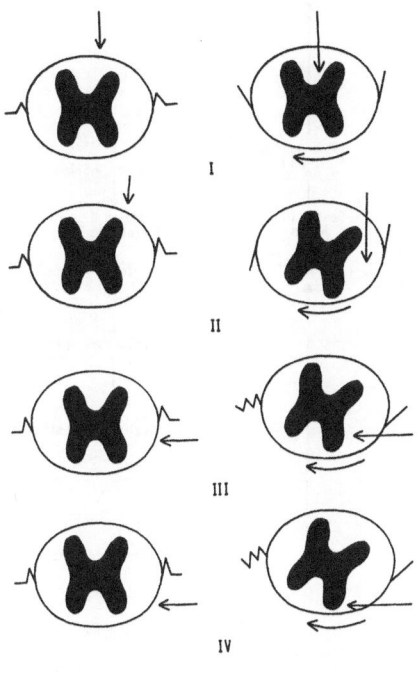

Fig. 3

cord is inevitable. Measurement of impedance and electrophysiological confirmation by the electrical stimulation, or by evoked potential, are therefore indispensable.

After aiming at the target according to the co-ordinates of the odontoid process and anterior and posterior surfaces of the cord visualized by Conray myelography, impedance and physiological responses are essential for confirmation of the site of electrode tip. Fig. 4 is an example of the physiological responses during cordotomy revealing not only the displacement of the surface of the cord (increase of impedance) but also the passive movement of the cord during the penetration of the electrode resulting in the prolongation of the diameter of the cord by 19 mm.

Using the postero-anterior track the responses from the dorsal fasciculus are good landmarks for confirmation of not only laterality but also depth of the electrode tip. As confirmed by many workers a "tingling" sensation of the caudal part of the body occurs with stimulation of the medial part of the fasciculus.

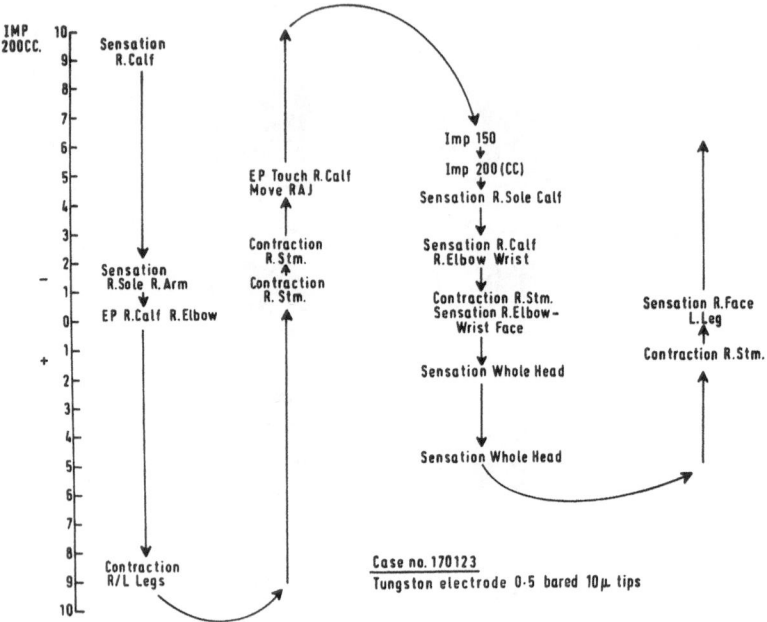

Fig. 4

The responses plotted from a patient treated by myelotomy are usually responses from the proximal part of the body that occur first (leg or arm) and gradually responses from distal parts (foot, hand, finger). This phenomenon is of interest anatomically as the somatotopic organisation in the dorso-ventral axis of the posterior fasciculus is still in dispute. Stimulation at the centre of the cord generally produces a burning sensation in the abdomen.

The somatotopic organization in the spinothalamic tract, revealed by plotting lateral tracts, confirms Walker's work[6], namely that the latero-posterior part represents the caudal part of the body. No difference was detected in the threshhold of electrical current and modality of responses between stimulation of the posterior fasciculi and the spinothalamic tract, the patient describing the sensation as either "tingling" or "pain" in each case.

In the spinothalamic tract the "spinal homonculus" appears to have a larger hand and foot than the posterior fasciculus homonculus.

Using these physiological methods the electrode is advanced or retracted or re-inserted until a response is obtained indicating correct positioning of the electrode tip. If this is achieved then only a relatively small coagulation (3 w 60 secs.) will achieve a satisfactory result.

References

1. Hitchcock, E. R. (1970), Stereotactic cervical myelotomy. J. Neurol. Neurosurg. Psychiat. *33*, 224—230.
2. — (1970), Stereotactic trigeminal tractotomy. Ann. Clin. Res. *2*, 131—135.
3. — (1972), Stereotaxis of the spinal cord. Confin. Neurol. *34*, 299—310.
4. Putman, T. J. (1934), Myelotomy of the commissure. Arch. Neurol. Psychiat. *32*, 1189—1193.
5. Taren, J. A., Davis, R., Crosby, E. C. (1969), Target physiologic corroboration in stereotactic cervical cordotomy. J. Neurosurg. *30*, 569—584.
6. Walker, A. E. (1940), The spinothalamic tract in man. Arch. Neurol. Psychiat. *43*, 284—298.

Authors' address: E. R. Hitchcock, M.D., and Y. Tsukamoto, M.D., Department of Surgical Neurology, Western General Hospital, Crewe Road, Edinburgh, Scotland.

Acta Neurochirurgica, Suppl. 21, 125—133 (1974)
© by Springer-Verlag 1974

Centre for Pain Relief, Liverpool Regional Department of Medical and
Surgical Neurology, Walton Hospital, Liverpool, England,
and Department of Mechanical Engineering, University of Salford, England

A Stereotactic Approach
to the Anterior Percutaneous Electrical Cordotomy

S. Lipton, E. Dervin, and O. B. Heywood

With 7 Figures

Introduction

The value of surgical cordotomy for the relief of intractable pain
was recognized by Spiller and Martin[2] in 1912, and by Foerster[1] 1913.
The percutaneous electrical cordotomy was introduced by Mullan[3, 4]
(1963, 1965) and modified by Rosomoff[5] (1965). This method, which
uses a lateral approach between C 1 and C 2, has the advantages of
avoiding major surgery and reducing mortality and morbidity.

The anterior approach technique was devised by Lin[6] (1966) to
avoid the dangers of "sleep apnoea" especially in patients requiring
bilateral operations. In this method the spinal needle traverses the
C 5/C 6 or neighbouring disc space and enters the dural sac from the
front. Lesions made at this level are below the outlet of the phrenic
nerve and the descending respiratory fibres are thus avoided.

If bilateral relief of pain is required either two anterior cordotomies
can be made or, alternatively, one anterior with one lateral at the
C 1/C 2 level where a high level of analgesia is needed on one side only.
The anterior cordotomy is also a safer procedure for the unilateral
treatment of pain in patients with poor lung function.

The percutaneous electrical cordotomy at the C 1/C 2 level is a relatively easy and well proven procedure using a lateral approach. However,
the anterior approach to the anterolateral tract through C 5/C 6 or
neighbouring disc space is a difficult freehand technique because the
track of the needle is predetermined by the geometry of the disc space.

The stereotactic method described is an attempt to overcome the
difficulties of the freehand anterior technique. The work is the result

of a joint project between the Department of Medical and Surgical Neurology, Walton Hospital, Liverpool and the Department of Mechanical Engineering of the University of Salford.

Problems of the Anterior Approach

In the anterior approach a target is selected on a line along a spinal tract (Fig. 1). It is the lateral (z) and anteroposterior (x) coordinates that are critical, the coordinate (y) along the target line is variable (Fig. 2).

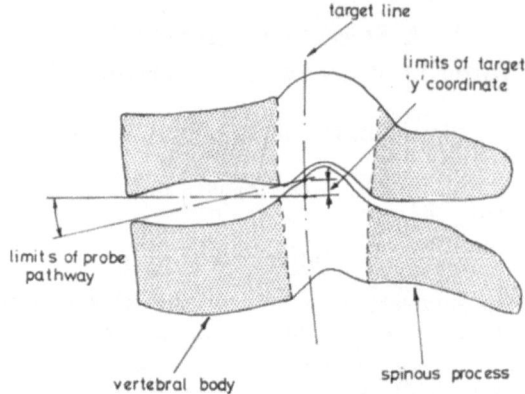

Fig. 1. Pathway limits through the disc space and the permissible variation of the target (y) coordinate

When an appropriate zone of entry to the intervertebral disc has been established a pathway through the disc has to be chosen which lies within the geometrical constraints imposed by the contours of the disc boundaries (Fig. 1). It is the determination of the compound angulation of this pathway which presents a major problem.

In the freehand technique the needle is inserted into the edge of the intervertebral disc, guided by an image intensifier.

An AP radiograph is used to determine the lateral displacement (z) of the needle tip from the target whilst the anteroposterior displacement (x) is determined from a lateral radiograph (Fig. 2).

The ratio z/x gives the tangent of the angle θ between the two planes.

(i) a vertical (sagittal) plane through the target,

(ii) a plane defined by the needle tip (P) and an axial line (YT) in the sagittal plane through the target (T).

The needle is then aligned into this plane by eye using a protractor or a Gildenberg[6] (1971) angle meter and then pushed through the disc to the target point still using the image intensifier for guidance.

This method of alignment by eye is difficult to achieve and the point of entry (P) may be inappropriate to reach the intended traget— i.e. the line PT may not be a possible pathway through the disc.

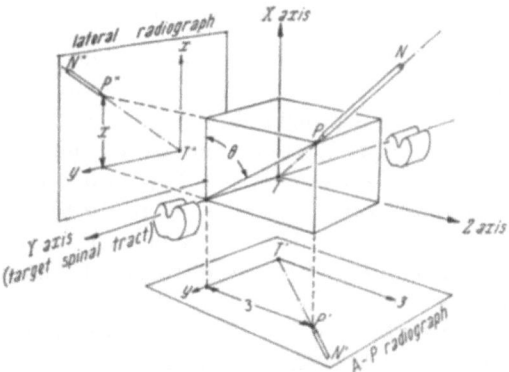

Fig. 2. Schematic drawing showing a section through the spinal cord and the angle θ which is obtained from the coordinates z and x on the lateral and antero-posterior radiographs respectively. It should be noted that this angle θ is not the true compound angle of the approach line (PT) to the vertical (X) axis

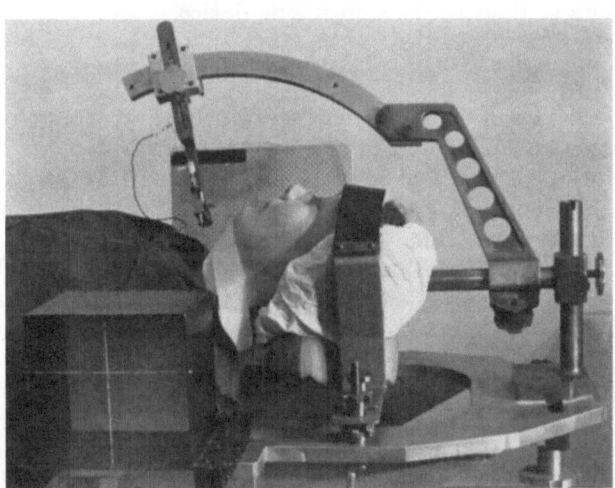

Fig. 3. The stereotactic device. The patient's head is positioned in an adjustable foam padded head-rest. The centre of the overhead bow can be adjusted in the x, y, and z directions by the movements incorporated in the post which carries the bow. The alignment device is shown in position for a lateral radiograph. Note the lead markers on the crosswires and on the plastic screen of the sighting box

The following stereotactic method eliminates the visual freehand alignment and provides a means of approaching a target along a cone of pathways with the correct point of entry to the disc located accordingly.

The Stereotactic Device

The system consists of a prefabricated aluminium base which replaces the head of the operating table. The base carries an overhead bow device, the centre of which can be adjusted in three dimensions to aim a needle at any chosen point (Fig. 3). Two angular movements incorporated in the bow device permit the needle to be aimed through the limited channel of pathways dictated by the geometry of the disc space. The use of an overhead bow of this type enables the operator to have a continuous view of the path of the needle (or electrode) using an image intensifier, because the axis of the bow does not obscure the radiographic field in either the lateral or antero-posterior projections (Fig. 3). The base frame also carries the X-ray film cassettes and the radiographic alignment devices necessary to establish the zero axes of the instrument, anatomical datum lines and the target coordinates. The patient's head is held firmly, not fixed, in a foam padded headrest. The purpose of the head rest is to help the patient to remain immobile whilst the two preliminary radiographs are taken to establish the x, y, and z settings of the stereotactic device.

Radiographic Alignment

The zero axes of the instrument are established by accurate alignment of the X-ray source and film relative to the base frame of the stereotactic device. A series of lead markers inserted in a perspex sheet is overlaid and positioned with the film cassette to provide reference axes on the radiograph (Fig. 4). Radiographic measurements are taken directly from the films using the constant magnification scale determined by the fixed distances between the X-ray source, anatomical target and film (Fig. 5).

The alignment method uses an optical technique consisting of sighting boxes with sets of cross markers (Fig. 3). The light beam from the optical delineator of the X-ray machine is used to project an image of the cross wires at the open end of the box onto a plastic screen. Correct alignment of the X-ray source with respect to the stereotactic instrument is achieved when the shadow of the cross wires is superimposed on the engraved cross of the plastic screen. The cross wires carry lead line markers which appear as dashes on the radiograph. Lead dot markers are inserted in the engraved cross of the plastic screen and also in the perspex overlay of the film. Correct alignment when the film is exposed

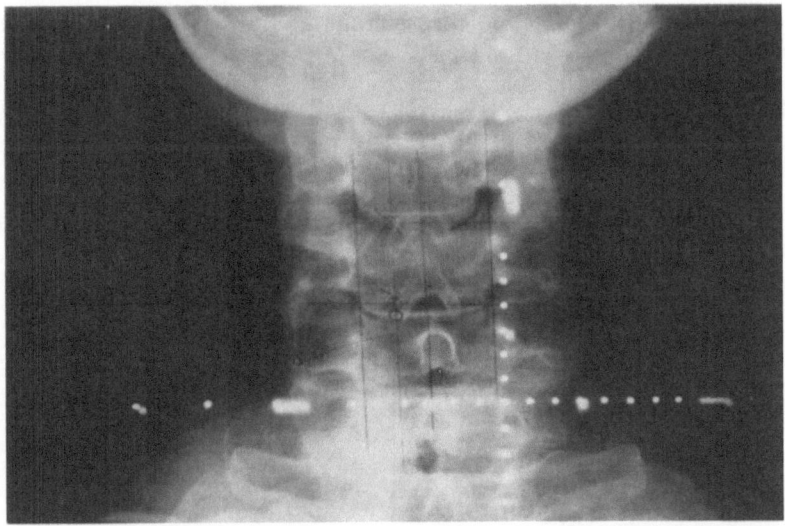

Fig. 4a. Preliminary antero-posterior radiograph. The lead markers of the radiographic alignment device and the film overlay are superimposed and show the correct alignment of the X-ray source and indicate the zero axes of the stereotactic instrument. The target line is also marked on the radiograph

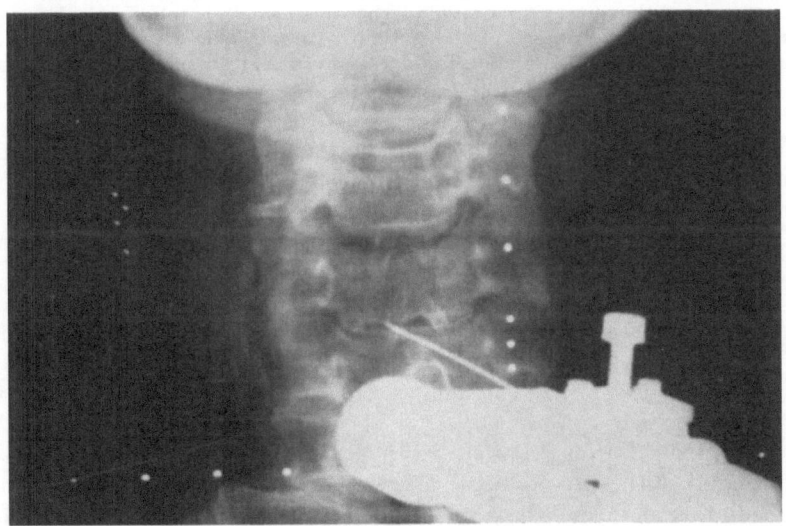

Fig. 4b. Stereotactic placement of the spinal needle to the target (antero-posterior radiograph)

is verified on the radiograph because the three sets of markers representing the three cross lines are superimposed (Fig. 4a). A simple distance
indicator between the X-ray tube and the sighting device maintains a
fixed distance and ensures constant magnification on the radiograph.

The Operating Procedure

(i) Patient lies in the supine position and is carefully aligned along
the centre line of the table and the stereotactic baseframe.

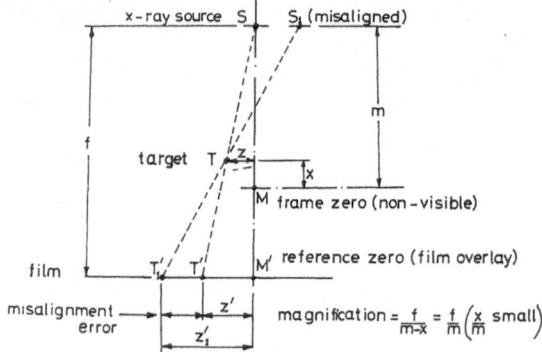

Fig. 5. Magnification and alignment problems. The magnification factor
is given by the ratio f/m provided that x is small, emphasising the need
for preliminary alignment of the patient's target structures. The possible
misalignment error $z_1' - z'$ is eliminated by correct alignment of the X-ray
source

(ii) The patient's head is fixed in the foam head-rest and the approximate position of the target line is adjusted by levelling screws in the
head holder to obtain known magnification on the radiograph.

(iii) Two radiographs are exposed using the careful alignment
techniques already described.

(iv) The target position is chosen on the radiographs and the instrument coordinate settings are read directly from the radiographs using
fixed magnification scales.

(v) The instrument coordinates are set and the needle holder is
fitted to the aiming bow.

(vi) Using the image intensifier the local anaesthetic needle is inserted
freehand to the pre-vertebral fascia and enters the disc space. The
orientation of this needle gives an indication of the angular settings of
the bow to allow the spinal needle to negotiate the disc space.

(vii) The stereotactic device is used to insert the spinal needle through
the disc space and its progress is checked by using the image intensifier.

If necessary the angular settings of the bow and needle carrier may be adjusted without jeopardising the target coordinates. It is also permissible to alter the non-critical y coordinate instrument setting if this is necessary to penetrate the disc space. If the patient is aligned correctly this manoeuver has little or no effect on the other two vital coordinates, namely the lateral (z) and the antero-posterior (x) settings (Fig. 2).

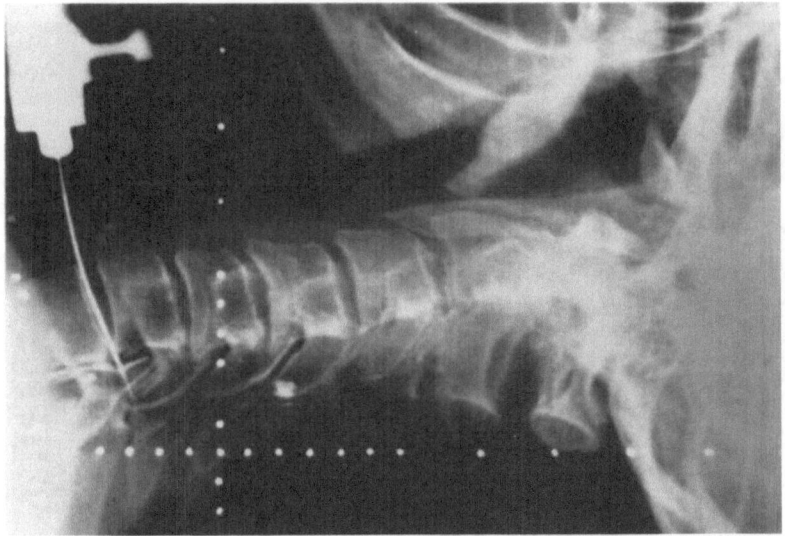

Fig. 6. Needle deflection in the lateral view. The lack of room for angulation of the needle is apparent in all the disc spaces

(viii) The final position of the needle is checked using normal stimulation procedures and impedance measurements. A lesion is made when a satisfactory target has been verified.

Clinical Results

Eighteen patients have been treated using the stereotactic device. Twelve procedures were completed with varying degrees of success. Six of the procedures were abandoned either because it was impossible to penetrate the diseased disc spaces (four cases) or there was insufficient room in the disc space and the pathway of the needle was deflected from its target (two cases, Figs. 6 and 7). In the twelve completed procedures, six of the patients were completely pain free until death, two patients had partial relief until death and four are counted as failures because the pain returned in periods varying from three days to two months.

Clinical experience has shown that two basic problems remain with the stereotactic apparatus.

(i) The deflection of the needle. At the present time there seems to be no complete answer to this problem. Preselection of patients for anterior cordotomy would certainly improve the rate of success. Patients should have an adequate disc space not only for passage of the needle but also to allow reasonable angulation of the needle within

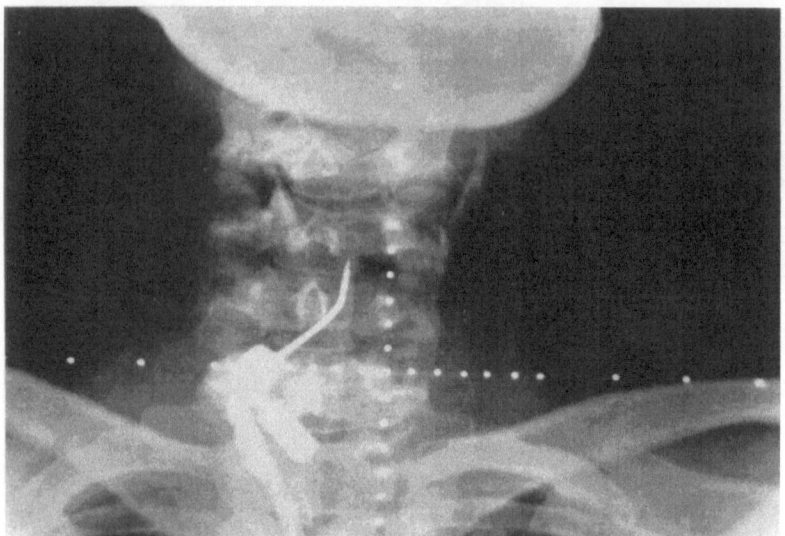

Fig. 7. Needle deflection in the antero-posterior view

the disc space. The length of the unsupported needle can also be reduced by elongating the needle carrier to the patient's neck.

(ii) Movement of the spinal structures relative to the external reference system. This could be reduced by replacing the foam head-rest with a pinion type of fixation device. This would also make it possible to rotate the head slightly and allow for better radiographic alignment of the mid-sagittal structures. However, this would be much more of an ordeal for the patient and would also lengthen the time taken for the procedure.

References

1. Foerster, O. (1913), Vorderseitenstrangdurchschneidung im Rücken-mark zur Beseitigung von Schmerzen. Berlin: Klin. Wschr. 50, 1499.
2. Spiller, W. G., Martin, E. (1912), The treatment of persistent pain of organic origin in the lower part of the body by division of the antero-lateral column of the spinal cord. J. Amer. med. Ass. 58, 1489—1490.

3. Mullan, S., Harper, P. V., Hekmatpanah, J., et al. (1963), Percutaneous interruption of spinal-pain tracts by means of a strontium[90] needle. J. Neurosurg. *20*, 931—940.
4. — Hekmatpanah, J., Dobben, G., Beckman, F. (1965), Percutaneous intramedullary cordotomy utilising the unipolar anodal electrolytic lesion. J. Neurosurg. *22*, 548—553.
5. Rosomoff, H. L., Carroll, F., Brown, J., et al. (1965), Percutaneous radiofrequency cervical cordotomy: technique. J. Neurosurg. *23*, 639—645.
6. Lin, P., Gildenberg, P. L., Polakoff, P. P. (1966), An anterior approach to percutaneous lower cervical cordotomy. J. Neurosurg. *25*, 553—560.
7. Gildenberg, P. L. (1971), Angle-meter to indicate the proper angle of insertion in anterior percutaneous cervical cordotomy. J. Neurosurg. *34*, 244—247.

Authors' addresses: S. Lipton, MB, ChB, FFRACS, Consultant Anaesthesist, Centre for Pain Relief, Liverpool Regional Department of Medical and Surgical Neurology, Walton Hospital, Liverpool, England, E. Dervin, BS (Tech), PhD, CEng, MIMechE., and O. B. Heywood, BSc (Eng), CEng, MIMechE., Lecturers in the Department of Mechanical Engineering, University of Salford, Salford M5 4 WT, Lancs., England.

Section III

Surgery of the Pituitary Gland and Hypothalamus

Acta Neurochirurgica, Suppl. 21, 137—143 (1974)

Departments of Clinical Surgery and Radiotherapy,
University of Edinburgh, Scotland

Pituitary Ablation by Yttrium-90

A. P. M. Forrest, M. M. Roberts, and H. J. Stewart

With 3 Figures

The method of pituitary ablation which we use is that of trans-phenoidal yttrium-screw implantation (Fig. 1) (Forrest, Blair, and Valentine, 1958). This modification of our original technique by which the yttrium rod is incorporated in a stainless steel screw unit was introduced to enable us to fix the radioactive source in an optimum position in the pituitary fossa (Forrest and Peebles Brown 1955, Forrest et al. 1956, Forrest et al. 1959).

This method has now been used to treat over 400 patients with advanced cancer of the breast. Of these, 387 treated between 1958 and December 1970 have been fully assessed. Their results will be used to illustrate several points of principle concerning this type of surgery in advanced cancer of the breast.

Selection of Patients

The selection of patients for pituitary ablation is best done within a defined policy of care. In our clinics it has generally been reserved for those premenopausal patients who initially have responded to oophorectomy and for postmenopausal patients who had initially been treated by simpler means—e.g. hormone therapy. In these circumstances it is used as an alternative to adrenalectomy, the choice being made on grounds of general fitness and type of disease. Women who have disseminated disease associated with a long "free interval", factors known to influence beneficially the response to endocrine surgery, are preferred for removal of the adrenals.

Technical Problems and Morbidity

For a fossa of normal size we have used a total activity of the sources of 10 mc in two yttrium rods. If the fossa is small, this is reduced. The activity must be checked locally before insertion.

We place the isotope at the junction of the lower and middle thirds of the fossa with the two units lying symmetrically close to the midline.

YTTRIUM-90 SCREW IMPLANTATION

OF THE PITUITARY

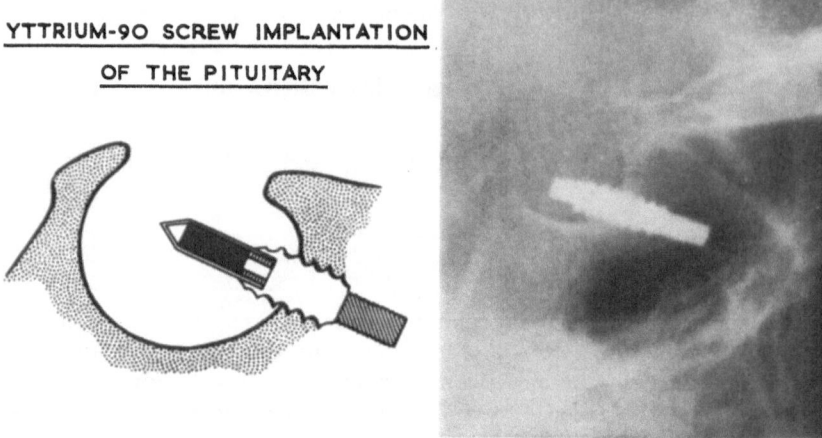

Fig. 1. Yttrium-90 screw implant, and implants in position

The morbidity of the procedure is due to irradiation damage to the roof of the fossa (if placed too high) or to its side walls (if placed too far from the midline). This may cause optic nerve damage, rhinorrhea and

Table 1. *Morbidity of Yttrium-90 Screw Implant in 387 Patients*

Meningitis	4.9%
Rhinorrhea total	5.2%
permanent	1.0%
Visual defects	1.8%
IIIrd nerve palsy	4.1%

meningitis or paralysis of the third, fourth and sixth nerves. Accurate assessment of morbidity must be made by the surgeon performing the operation. Only too frequently this is not done. As a result, referring physicians accept that the procedure gives benefit without true knowledge of its risks.

All our patients have been regularly followed-up by one of our team. The morbidity statistics are given in Table 1.

Completeness of Hypophysectomy

The aim of pituitary implantation is to suppress completely pituitary function. Yet many authors, when describing their technique, omit any reference to the extent of destruction they achieve. The *anatomical extent* of destruction is the most exact measurement but this can be assessed only post mortem. In our experience 40% of 77 patients who

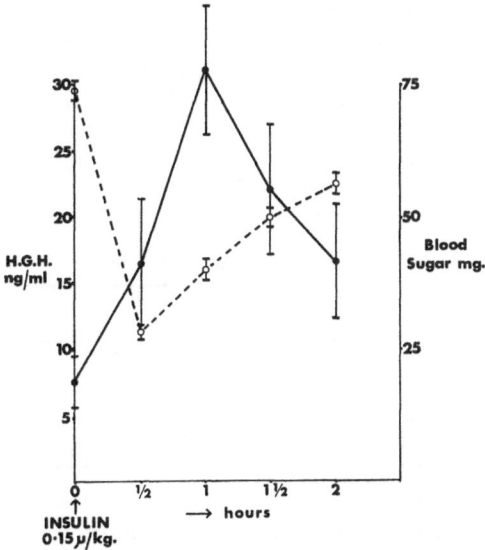

Fig. 2. Growth hormone response to insulin induced hypoglycaemia

had multiple sections of the pituitary fossa examined by Dr. A. T. Sandison (Glasgow) post mortem had pituitary remnants which were estimated to exceed 15% of the gland volume.

Functional evidence of destruction, although more difficult to assess, is of greater value in the management of the patient. We have found the growth hormone response to insulin hypoglycaemia the most convenient test (Stewart et al. 1970). The form of the test is shown in Fig. 2. An increment of 4 ng or more in the plasma growth hormone level following the production of adequate hypoglycaemia by 0.1 units of insulin/kg intravenously is taken as positive evidence of incomplete ablation. It is our practice to perform this test three months after implantation. To date, 9 of the 49 patients thus studied have had a positive response.

From these considerations it would appear that the pituitary continues to function following implantation in approximately one-fifth of patients.

Assessment of Clinical Response

The assessment of the clinical response to hypophysectomy, whichever method is used, must be critical and objective. This demands careful and full documentation of the patient at each attendance and a decision by more than one person of the clinical response.

Like others with experience of this disease, we now use a system which categorises objective responses in three ways: clear cut (when all metastatic lesions have regressed); failure (when all lesions are progressing) and equivocal (when there is doubt—some lesions apparently improving, others remaining static). Details of our assessment and those used in other centres are to be found in the Second Tenovus Workshop (1970). Our results in 274 patients in whom such assessment has been possible are shown in Table 2.

Table 2. *Remission Rates (%) in 274 Assessable Patients*

Remission	All patients	"Fit" patients
Clear cut	15.3	18.5
Equivocal	8.8	9.3
Total	24.1	27.8

A true assessment of the value of implantation can be made only by comparison with another standard method of treatment. This we have done in two controlled randomised studies, recently reported by Roberts (1970).

The first, in Glasgow, was designed to compare yttrium-90 screw implantation with adrenalectomy and oophorectomy. Seventy-six patients were included between 1958 and 1962, all with metastatic cancer of the breast. Thirty-seven were treated by yttrium implant and 39 by adrenalectomy and oophorectomy. All now are dead. The incidence of remission was similar in the two groups but the duration of remission was longer, but not significantly so, in those treated by yttrium implant. The duration of survival of those patients who responded was significantly greater in the patients treated by adrenalectomy but not so when all patients in the two groups were considered (Table 3).

The second trial, in Cardiff, compared yttrium-90 implant with transethmoidal hypophysectomy. One hundred and one patients were included and treated between 1966 and 1969. The transethmoidal hypophysectomies were carried out by Mr. Stephen Richards. All but 6 of these 101 patients are now dead. Although the incidence of remission

Table 3. *Comparison of Yttrium-90 Screw Implant and Adrenalectomy and Oophorectomy in 76 Patients with Metastatic Cancer of the Breast*

Figures marked with an asterisk are significantly different

	No. of patients	Remission rate (%)		Duration in responders (weeks)		Mean survival of those dead in total groups (weeks)
		Clear cut	Equivocal	Remission	Survival	
90Y implant	37	22	15	50.1	90.6*	50.8
Adrenalectomy + oophorectomy	39	24	12	100.9	153.1*	175.4

Table 4. *Comparison of Yttrium-90 Screw Implant and Transethmoidal Hypophysectomy in 101 Patients with Metastatic Cancer of the Breast*

Figures marked with an asterisk are significantly different

	No. of patients	Remission rate (%)		Duration in responders (weeks)		Mean survival of those dead in total groups (weeks)
		Clear cut	Equivocal	Remission	Survival	
90Y implant	50	28	4	49.9*	97.6	47.2
Transethmoidal hypophysectomy	51	12	6	106.2*	122.2	51.5

was higher in those treated by yttrium implant, the duration of remission was significantly longer in those who responded to transethmoidal hypophysectomy. Survival in those patients who responded to transethmoidal hypophysectomy also was longer, but the cumulative survival curves of all patients admitted to the trial were uninfluenced by the treatment group to which they had been allocated (Fig. 3) (Table 4).

In this trial, 52 patients had a growth hormone-insulin test three months after surgery. The incidence of positive responses was 28%

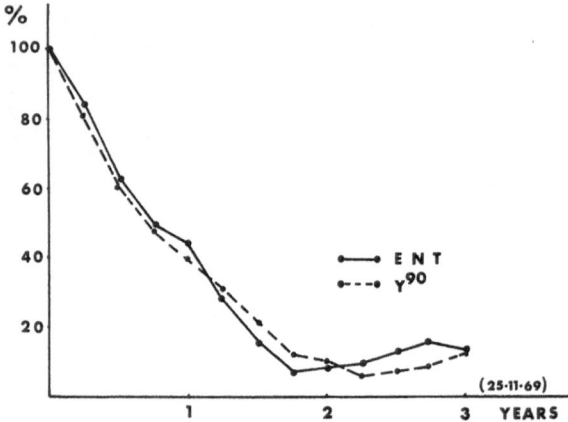

Fig. 3. Cumulative survival curves of 101 patients with metastatic breast cancer randomly treated by Yttrium-90 screw implant or transethmoidal hypophysectomy

of 25 patients in the transethmoidal group and 11% of 27 patients treated by yttrium implant.

Our studies indicate that neither yttrium-90 screw implantation of the pituitary nor transethmoidal hypophysectomy regularly achieves complete destruction of the gland. We believe that this accounts for our finding that adrenalectomy and oophorectomy give slightly superior results. This is in contrast to the reported results of transfrontal hypophysectomy. The long term results of a trial in Guys Hospital, which was designed to compare transfrontal hypophysectomy and adrenalectomy, now indicate that the former operation is better (Hayward 1970). Nevertheless, yttrium-90 implant and other stereotactic methods of suppressing pituitary function have the value of simplicity and of causing little upset to the patient. Therefore it is particularly suitable for the ill patient and those in whom other more radical forms of endocrine ablation are not considered justified.

References

Forrest, A. P. M., Peebles Brown, D. A. (1955), Pituitary-radon implant for breast cancer. Lancet 2, 1054—1055.
— — Morris, S. R., Illingworth, D. F. W. (1956), Pituitary-radon implant for advanced cancer. Lancet 1, 399—401.
— Blair, D. W., Valentine, J. S. (1958), Screw implantation of the pituitary with yttrium-90. Lancet 2, 192—193.
— — Peebles Brown, D. A., Stewart, H. J., Sandison, A. T., Harrington, R. W., Valentine, J. M., Carter, P. T. (1959), Radio-active implantation of the pituitary. Brit. J. Surg. 47, 61—70.
Hayward, J. L. (1970), Second Tenovus Workshop. Clinical trials comparing transfrontal hypophysectomy with adrenalectomy and with transethmoidal hypophysectomy. In: The clinical management of advanced breast cancer, p. 50. Eds. C. A. F. Joslin and E. N. Gleave. Cardiff: Alpha Omega Publishing Co.
Roberts, M. M. (1970), Second Tenovus Workshop. A comparison of transethmoidal hypophysectomy, yttrium-90 implant and adrenalectomy. In: The clinical management of advanced breast cancer, p. 54. Eds. C. A. F. Joslin and E. N. Gleave. Cardiff: Alpha Omega Publishing Co.
Second Tenovus Workshop (1970), The clinical management of advanced breast cancer. Eds. C. A. F. Joslin and E. N. Gleave. Cardiff: Alpha Omega Publishing Co.
Stewart, H. J., Benson, E. A., Roberts, M. M., Forrest, A. P. M., Greenwood, F. C. (1970), Pituitary function after yttrium implants as measured by plasma growth hormone levels. J. Endocr. 50, 41—50.

Authors' address: Prof. A. P. M. Forrest, Department of Clinical Surgery, Royal Infirmary, Lauriston Place, Edinburgh EH3 9YW, Scotland.

Acta Neurochirurgica, Suppl. 21, 145—149 (1974)
© by Springer-Verlag 1974

Hypophysectomy—The Combined Role of Neuro- and Rhino-Surgeons

J. Angell-James

The hypophysis being situated in the zone that separates the field of the neuro from that of the rhino surgeon, has interested both specialties for many years, encouraged by the pioneer work of Cushing (1912) and Hirsch (1952), Cushing in the first specialty and Hirsch in the second. For many years, however, the neurosurgical transfrontal approach has dominated the scene.

Three factors have led to a return of interest in the trans-sphenoidal operation:

1. The application of micro-surgery to rhinology following the improvements in equipment and the training of all otolaryngologists in this technique.

2. The introduction of antibiotics, which dramatically reduced the hazards of meningitis as a complication.

3. The developement of hormone ablation surgery, requiring removal of the normal gland in a very considerable number of patients in poor condition for such diseases as metastatic breast cancer.

The advantages of the trans-sphenoidal route are that:

1. The operation is short, usually 45 minutes, with minimal shock.

2. The sella can be visualized directly and fully with the binocular operating microscope.

3. The haemorrhage is easily controllable.

4. There is no disturbance of the brain.

5. Post operative discomfort is minimal.

There are, however, certain disadvantages, the most important of which are:

1. Nasal sepsis which cannot be eliminated. This is an absolute contraindication, but in the author's series it has been possible to eliminate it even in patients with active chronic sinusitis.

2. Lack of pneumatisation of the sphenoidal sinuses, which is found in approximately 3 per cent of patients.

Advances   10

Total Operations—401

Mammary carcinoma (female)	343
Mammary carcinoma (male)	2
Diabetic retinopathy	20
Prostatic carcinoma	14
Malignant melanoma	7
Acromegaly	8
Chromophobe edenoma	4
Cushing's syndrome	1
Granulosa cell tumour of the ovary	1
Ovarian carcinoma	1

Complications of Hypophysectomy in the Early Group of 258 Operations

Meningitis	13
C.S.F. leakage	32
Persistent anosmia	8
Immediate diabetes insipidus	129
Operative haemorrhage	15
Excessive weight gain	8
Unilateral blindness	2

Complications Last 100 Cases

Cerebro spinal leak	1
Ocular palsy	0
Meningitis	1

Post-Operative Mortality—Total 8% in Last 100 Cases

Directly attributable to the operation:

    1 Cortisone crisis   1%

Attributable to the disease:

    2 Pulmonary metastases
    2 Pulmonary embolism
    1 Intestinal metastasis
      with haemorrhage   7%
    1 Abdominal perforation
    1 Hepatic metastases

Mammary Cancer—343 Cases

Survival after Hypophysectomy	
Months	Number surviving
6	174
12	106
18	63
24	42
30	27
36	22
42	13
48	8
54	7
60	6
66	4
72	3
78	2
84	1

Duration of Remission or Arrest—343 Cases

Months	Number	Percentage
1	242	70
3	192	55
6	110	31
9	86	25
12	70	21
18	37	11
24	27	8
36	8	4
48	4	2
60	3	1
72	1	0.3
84	1	0.3

3. Abnormal development of the cavernous sinuses towards the midline in the dura lining the anterior wall of the sella rendering the final opening of the capsule somewhat difficult.

4. Post operative cerebro-spinal fluid leak, with attendant risk of meningitis.

Of the trans-sphenoidal routes of access, the two most popular are the trans-ethmoidal, described by Chiari (1912) and the trans-antral, popularized by Hamberger (1961). The author favours the trans-ethmoidal route because it is the shorter, the more direct, the less traumatic, and does not involve the mouth (James, J. Angell 1965). It also has the important advantage of working along the line of the cribriform plate, which is the second of the two main sites from which cerebro-spinal fluid leak can occur, the other site being the diaphragma sellae.

The Technique of the Transethmo-sphenoidal Operation

A curved incision is made over the lateral aspect of the nose, anterior to the lacrimal sac and the internal tarsal ligament. The orbital periosteum is elevated and the anterior ethmoidal artery is coagulated. The ethmoidal cells are excised as far as is necessary to expose the full extent of the anterior surface of the sphenoid bone. The posterior third of the nasal septum is fenestrated to provide access to the sphenoidal sinus on the opposite side. The anterior wall of the sphenoidal sinuses is fenestrated. The dura covering the gland is exposed by fenestrating the bony posterior wall of the sinuses. The dura is incised with diathermy employing a cruciate incision. The gland is then dissected free with special dissectors and removed with fenestrated forceps. Meticulous removal of all final fragments is important if the best result is to be obtained. This is the most difficult part of the operation because the gland is often very soft. The final most important step is to seal off the operculum in the diaphragm with a disc of fascia lata held in place by a muscle pack, firmly rammed into the sella, and finally the placement of a fascia lata patch over the window. This is firmly packed and retained in place with an absorbable ribbon gauze pack, threaded with nylon and impregnated with sulphonamides and antibiotics or antiseptics. The remains of the pack are removed at the end of a week.

Results

During the last 12 years 401 operations have been performed. The results were marred in the earlier years by the frequency of post operative cerebro-spinal leak, but in the last 100 operations, there has only been one case in which a temporary leak of two or three days may have occurred. There has also been one case of meningitis, which occurred in spite of the absence of any C.S.F. leak. Recovery took place after antibiotic treatment, lumbar puncture and intrathecal antibiotics.

Discussion

The trans-frontal approach will always be indicated for tumours with large suprasellar extensions, but for hormone ablation and many of the smaller tumours, the trans-sphenoidal approach provides all the access that is necessary for safe and thorough surgery.

When the main tumour is intrasellar, even if it is quite large, the trans-sphenoidal operation is very much easier than the majority of operations for removal of the normal gland, because the cavernous sinuses are compressed laterally and a very large avascular window is available for access to the sella. The intra-cranial pressure tends to force the upper extensions of the tumour downwards into the sella as the lower intra-sellar portion is removed, and thus complete removal of most tumours is technically possible by this route.

This field of surgery is ideally one which should be handled by a combined team of neuro and rhino surgeons, working in close co-operation. It may well be argued that a number of neurosurgeons are also expert in rhino-surgery, but the rhino surgeon has, by training and practice, exceptional skills and facility in operating with the microscope in the restricted field of the nasal sinuses, and it is by taking advantage of this expertise that the finest results can be achieved.

References

1. Chiari, O. (1912), Über eine Modifikation der Schlofferschen Operation von Tumoren der Hypophyse. Wien. klin. Wschr. *25*, 5—6.
2. Cushing, H. (1912), The pituitary body and its disorders. Philadelphia: Lippincott.
3. Hamberger, C. A., Hammer, G., Norlen, G., Sjorgren, B. (1961), Transantrosphenoidal hypophysectomy. Arch. Otolaryng. (Chicago) *74*, 2—8.
4. Hirsch, A. (1952), Symptoms and treatment of pituitary tumors. A. M. A. Arch. of Otolar. *55*, 268—306.
5. Hirsch, A. (1956), Hypophysentumoren — Ein Grenzgebiet. Acta Neurochir. *5*, 1—10.
6. Angell-James, J. (1967), The Semon Lecture "The Hypophysis". J. Laryng. Otol. *81*, 1283—1307.

Author's address: J. Angell-James, Litfield House, Clifton Down, Bristol, England.

Acta Neurochirurgica, Suppl. 21, 151—158 (1974)
© by Springer-Verlag 1974

The Radiodiagnostic Department and the Section of Neurological Science,
The London Hospital, London E 1 1 BB, England

Radiological Assessment of the Pituitary Gland

L. Morris and I. Wylie

With 8 Figures

Introduction

The treatment of pituitary gland tumours, particularly where there is no clinical evidence of supra-sellar extension, rarely involves an open surgical procedure. In these cases, pituitary ablation can be carried out by one of several methods including trans-sphenoidal and trans-ethmoidal hypophysectomy, trans-sphenoidal cryosurgery, trans-sphenoidal yttrium implantation, external irradiation and transfrontal stereotactic yttrium implantation. Irrespective of the method employed, accurate investigation of the pituitary gland is essential, but this is particularly important with stereotactic implantation.

Method

It is necessary to determine the volumetric size of the gland, the limits of its extent and the presence or otherwise of asymmetrical growth within the sella. It is also necessary to exclude the possibility that some other structure (i.e. of a non-pituitary nature) is contributing to the contents of the sella. To this end, it is necessary to carry out:

1) plain film examination of the skull, including coronal and sagittal tomography of the pituitary fossa;
2) lumbar pneumoencephalography;
3) bilateral carotid arteriography;
4) cavernous sinus venography.

Apart from the first of these, the order in which the contrast procedures are carried out is not important. In addition, it is possible to exclude from the first examination tomography of the pituitary fossa if it has already been decided that pneumoencephalography will be carried out for the reason that tomography of this area forms part of a pneumoencephalographic examination. The first three examinations listed are already well established as routine pre-operative investigations (Cross et al. 1972). These will therefore not be discussed in detail except to stress certain features relevant to these examinations.

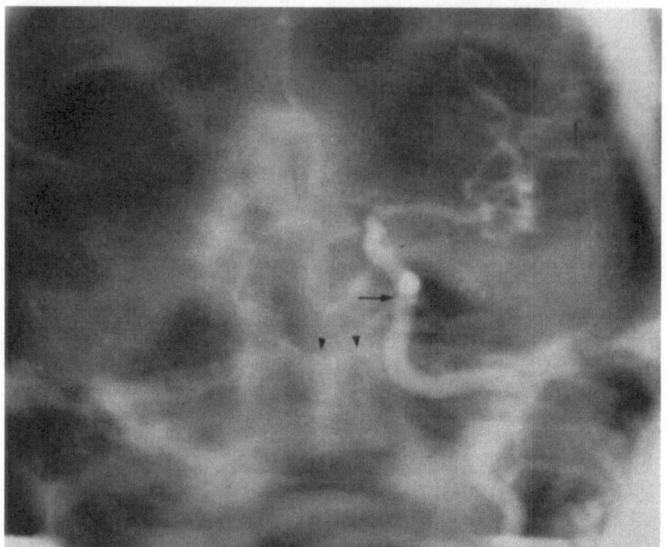

Fig. 1. Frontal angio-tomography during carotid arteriography. There is lateral displacement of the carotid siphon (arrow) and downward displacement of the floor of the sella (arrow heads)

Bilateral carotid angiography: This will demonstrate the relationship of the carotid siphons to the sella, and a rough estimation can be made of possible lateral extension of the pituitary gland, as indicated by widening of the loops of the carotid siphon and lateral displacement of the siphon away from the mid-line. This can be carried out in the routine way, but clarification of the position of the carotid siphon may be obtained by the use of angio-tomography (Fig. 1). Equally important is to exclude the possibility that any part of the fossa is occupied by the carotid siphon itself so that this structure can be avoided during the surgical procedure (Fig. 2). The presence of internal carotid aneurysm can also be excluded.

Pneumoencephalography: It is essential during the pneumoencephalographic examination to obtain sagittal and frontal tomography of the sella and the gas-filled subarachnoid cisterns in relation to it. By this means the bony margins of the sella can be assessed and the diaphragmae sellae and the optic nerves and chiasm can be accurately identified. The importance of this has been previously stressed by McLachlan, Lavender, and Edwards (1971). The apparatus used in the present study (Diagnost N—Philips) has a constant magnification factor of 1 : 1.3, so that the parameters of the pituitary gland and the distance of the

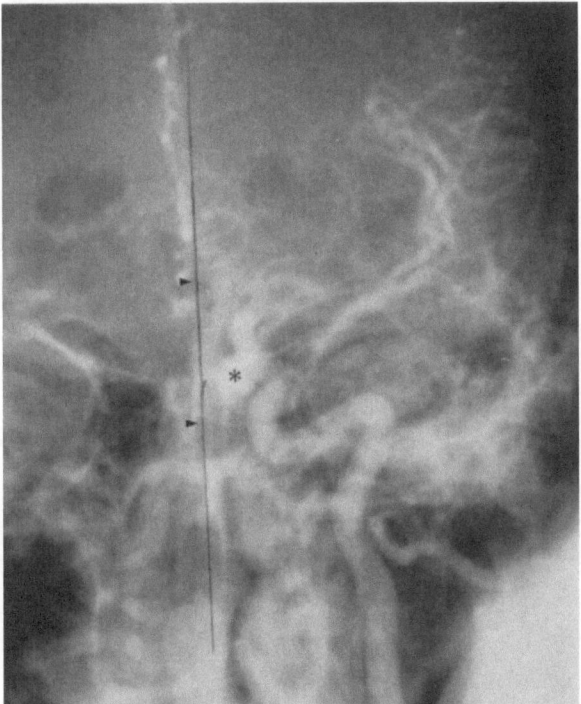

Fig. 2. Carotid arteriography demonstrating that a loop of the carotid siphon (*) extends into the pituitary fossa and reaches almost to the midline (arrow heads)

optic nerves and chiasm from identifiable anatomical points of the pituitary gland and fossa can be accurately measured (Figs. 3, 4, and 5). With this information it is possible to achieve precise implantation of the radioactive substance and avoid unnecessary irradiation of the optic nerves and chiasm. At this stage of the examination it is possible to demonstrate whether or not there is any prolongation of the chiasmatic cistern into the sella itself, the so-called "empty sella" syndrome (Kaufman 1968). This is particularly important when the trans-sphenoidal approach is being used.

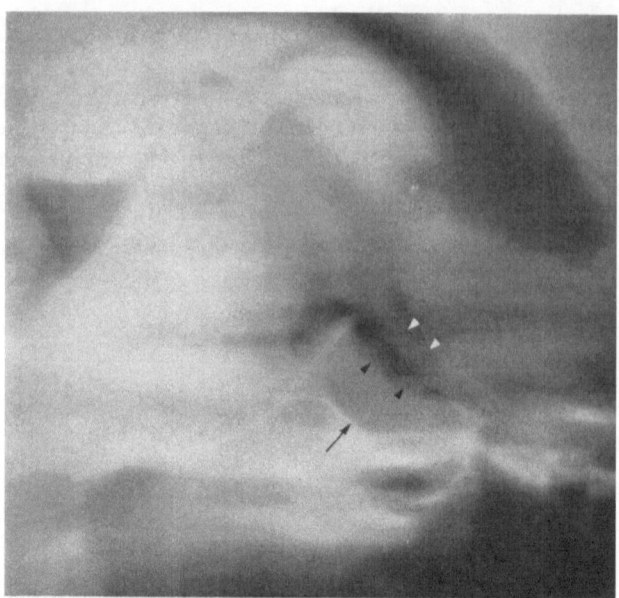

Fig. 3. Mid-line sagittal tomogram during encephalography, demonstrating an enlarged sella. The optic nerves (white arrow heads) are seen and the distance from the bony sella and diaphragmae (black arrow heads) can be measured. The sella floor is seen (arrow)

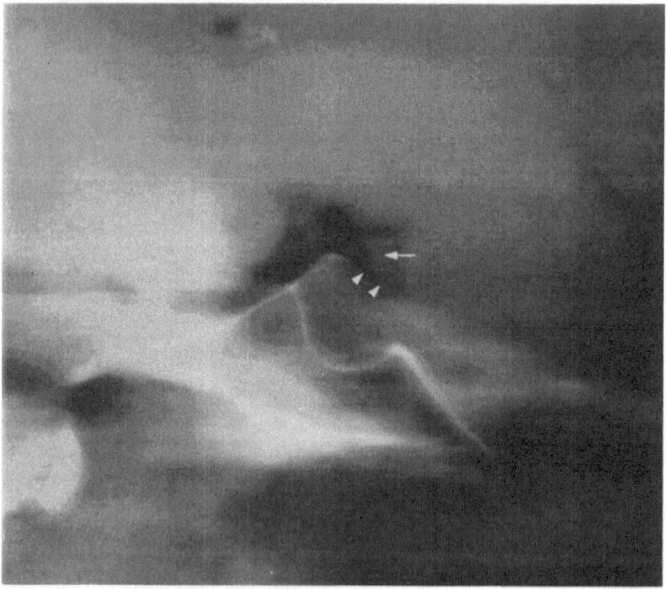

Fig. 4. Mid-line sagittal tomogram during encephalography demonstrating the optic nerves (arrow) and showing sella enlargement with some upward extension of the diaphragmae (arrow heads)

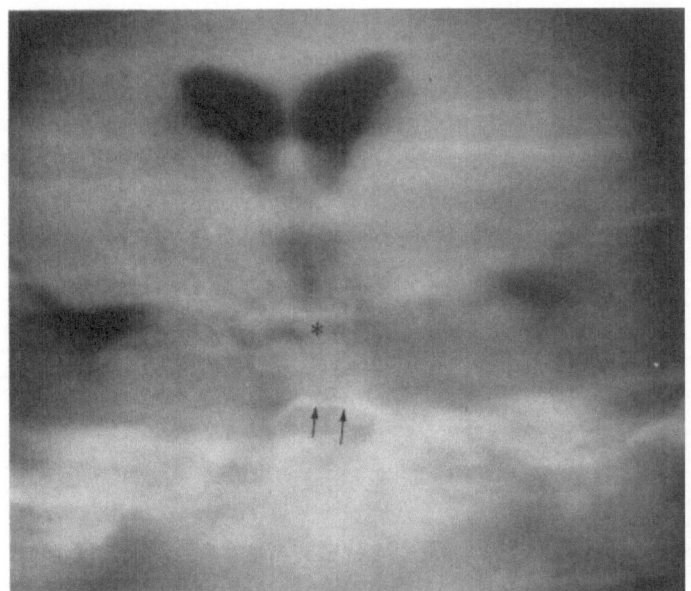

Fig. 5. Coronal tomogram during pneumoencephalography showing a tilt of the floor of the sella (arrows) and demonstrating the chiasmatic cistern (*)

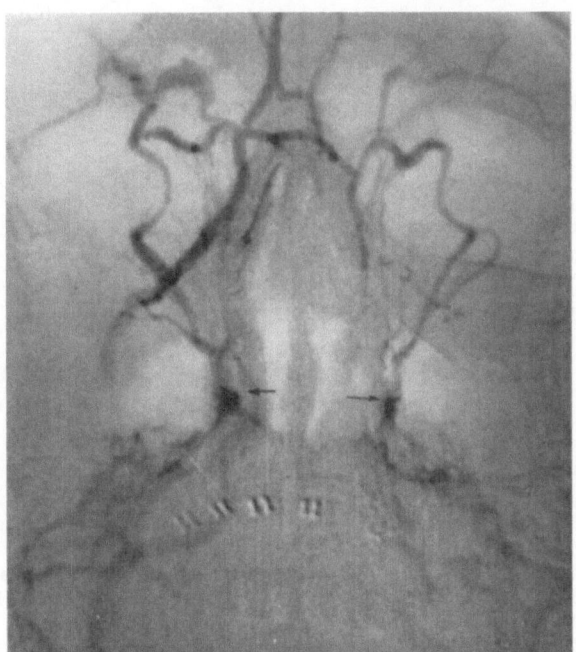

Fig. 6. Semi-axial view during orbital venography. Subtraction film. The cavernous sinuses are demonstrated (arrows). These are displaced laterally, more particularly the left

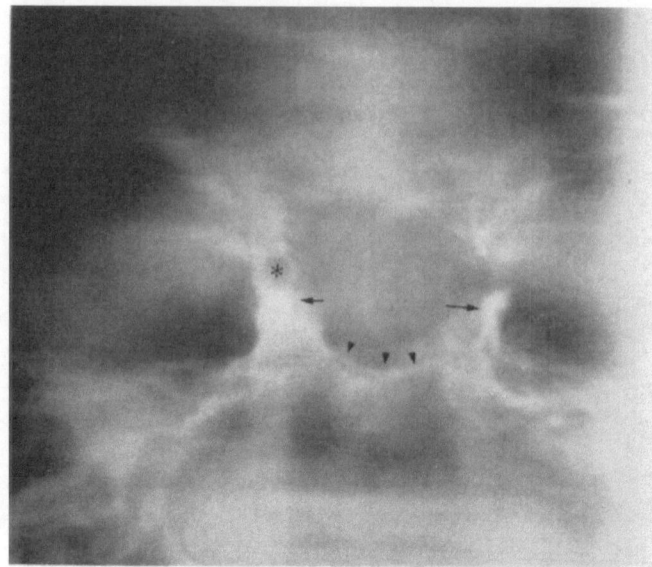

Fig. 7. Coronal tomogram through the pituitary fossa and cavernous sinus during venography. The floor of the sella is depressed (arrow heads). Both cavernous sinuses show some lateral displacement but particularly the left (arrows). The negative shadow of the carotid artery is clearly seen (*)

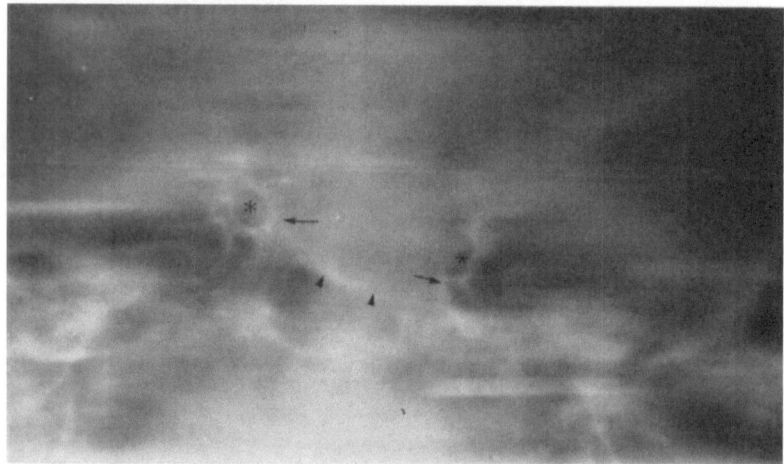

Fig. 8. Coronal tomography during frontal venography. The cavernous sinuses (arrows) are displaced laterally by the pituitary tumour. The negative shadows of the carotid siphons are seen within the cavernous sinuses (*). The floor of the sella is depressed (arrow heads)

Cavernous sinus venography: Carotid arteriography is a relatively crude method of demonstrating lateral extension of the pituitary gland as displacement of the intra-cavernous portions of the carotid artery probably only occur in relatively large tumours. Pneumoencephalography is of limited value in the demonstration of lateral extension of the pituitary gland as the cavernous sinus and its contents intervene between the pituitary gland and the gas-filled subarachnoid spaces. Assessment of the width of the bony floor of the sella is similarly of only limited value in determination of lateral extension of the gland. Lloyd (1972) has shown that satisfactory demonstration of the cavernous sinuses can be obtained by frontal vein injection of contrast medium and using subtraction techniques (Fig. 6). This will give a good assessment of the medial borders of the cavernous sinuses and give a more accurate assessment of lateral extension of the pituitary gland than does carotid arteriography. To this we have added the use of coronal angiotomography during frontal venography, and this, in addition to confirming lateral displacement of the cavernous sinus, allows us to measure the inter-sinus distance with a high degree of accuracy (Figs. 7 and 8). Here again, for practical purposes, the films show a magnification of 1 : 1.3.

Using all the measurements thus obtained and applying the formula $H/2 \times L/2 \times W/2 \times 4/3 \times 11$, assuming the shape of the pituitary gland is ellipsoid, we can then estimate the volume of the pituitary gland (Di Chiro 1960).

Summary

Routine procedures in the assessment of pituitary gland size and shape, supplemented by more sophisticated manoeuvres, have enabled us to provide the surgeon with extremely accurate information as to the dimensions of the gland and the extent of its extra-sellar extension. This has been useful in guiding the surgeon during stereotactic yttrium implantation into the pituitary gland.

References

1. Cross, J. N., Gynne, A., Grossart, K. W. M., Jennett, W. B., Kellett, R. J. (1972), Treatment of acromegaly by cryosurgery. Lancet *I*, 215—216.

2. Di Chiro, G. (1960), The width (third dimension) of the sella turcica. Amer. J. Roentgenol. Rad. Therapy and Nucl. Med. *84*, 26—37.

3. Kaufman, B. (1968), The empty sella turcica—a manifestation of the intra-sellar subarachnoid space. Radiology *28*, 351—356.

4. Lloyd, G. A. S. (1972), The localisation of lesions in the orbital apex and cavernous sinus by frontal venography. Brit. J. Radiol. *45*, 405—414.

5. McLachlan, M. S. F., Lavender, J. P., Edwards, C. R. W. (1971), Poly-tome-encephalography in the investigation of pituitary tumours. Clin. Radiol. *22*, 361—369.

Authors' address: L. Morris, M.D., and I. Wylie, M.D., The London Hospital, London E 1 1 BB, England.

Acta Neurochirurgica, Suppl. 21, 159—163 (1974)
© by Springer-Verlag 1974

Department of Stereotactic Neurosurgery, Psychiatric Hospital, Santiago,
Chile

Stereotactic Pituitary Implantation of Radioisotopes by Transfrontal Route

300 Cases

M. Poblete and R. Zamboni

With 2 Figures

Several procedures for hypophysectomy have been reported during the last years[1, 6, 4, 3]. All of them have been conceived to simplify surgery as much as possible. This is understandable by the fact that they are performed upon patients with diseases which often involve their general condition and surgical stress must be reduced to a minimum.

Hypophyseal interstitial irradiation placing Yttrium-90 pellets trans-nasally in the sella turcica is one of the methods most frequently used[6, 3, 10]. But the need of general anesthesia, the risk of CSF fistula and the possibility of infection moved us to use the transfrontal route.

Apart from Riechert and Mundinger's original work[9] and our own[5], we have not been able to find other publications regarding this technique and so we find useful its reactualization.

Our experience is based in 300 procedures: 201 for advanced breast cancer, 25 for prostatic carcinoma, 39 for acromegaly, 13 for diabetic retinopathy and 22 cases with miscellaneous diagnosis in whom hypo-physectomy was indicated.

Our results are comparable to those of other authors using different techniques and hence will not be discussed.

The purpose of this report is to review the operative technique and to analyse the complications and advantages of this procedure.

Technique

With the patient in face-up position, premedicated with Fentanyl (R) and Droperidol (R), the Riechert and Mundinger stereotactic apparatus is placed below the sellar floor plane. On the A-P film the target point is marked in the midline. On the lateral view the target point is placed in the anterior portion of the sella, more than 3 mm below the inter-clinoidal plane and more than 2 mm above the floor.

The puncture trajectory is calculated with an angle of 35 to 40 degrees in relation to the anterior fossa. This allows the subsequent introduction without problems of an instrument between the anterior border of the chiasm and the tuberculum sellae, considering the posterior chiasmatic position to be the most frequent. Through a right frontal trephine

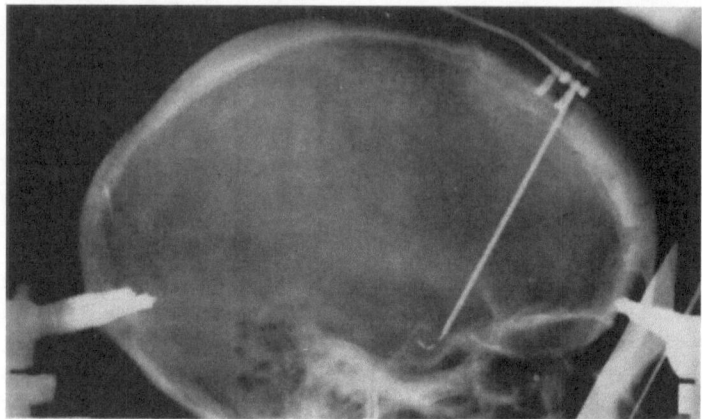

Fig. 1. Radiographic control of inactive pellets

(at 2 cm from the midline) a trocar of 1.2 mm diameter is introduced under television monitoring. Usually the sellar diaphragma offers a slight resistance. At this moment the patient has pain of mild intensity, referred to the glabella or bitemporal areas. In the few cases in which the chiasm is in an anterior position, a characteristic elastic resistance is felt with the cannula. In this cases it is necessary to modify the angle of the puncture trajectory to 50 degrees in order to reach the sella behind the posterior border of the chiasm. Once the cannula has reached the target point, two inactive pellets of Yttrium-90 are deposited and the instrument is withdrawn up to the interclinoidal plain (Fig. 1). This is to verify that later the radioactive material will not be subject to any movements when actual implantation is performed. In the few cases in which the control pellets show displacement, it is sufficient to deepen the cannula 0.5 to 1 mm in order to avoid it. After satisfactory antero-posterior and lateral control films are obtained the active 1×1.5 mm pellets are deposited under visual control. The radioactive dose used to obtain total destruction of the pituitary is 15 mC (100,000 rads at the periphery) distributed in about 8 pellets (Fig. 2). A peripheral dose of 20,000 rads from Yttrium-90 source was used when partial hypo-pituitarism was desirable. In cases with eosinophilic tumours and a large sella turcica, an additional dose of 5000 to 10,000 rads from Iridium-192 source was added[7]. Iridium-192 was used as 0.3 mm diameter wire with a length according to its specific activity.

After surgery penicillin is used during the first three days. Treatment with cortisone (37 mg) is started at the third day.

Pituitary function is evaluated by urinary gonadotrophines test and

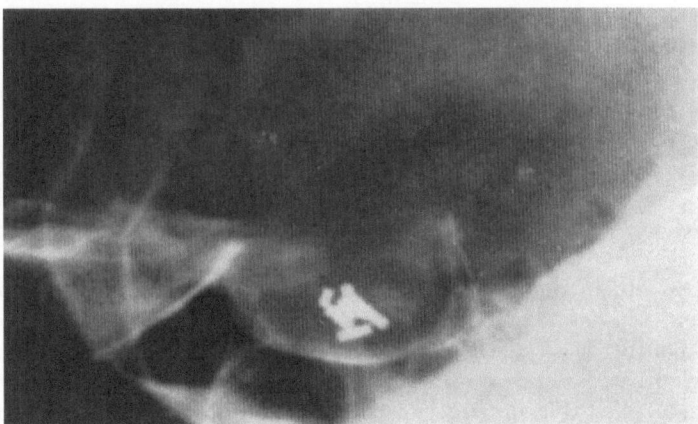

Fig. 2. Radiographic control of position of pellets (lateral view)

iodine thyroid-131 uptake, pre-operatively and about thirty days after surgery. When hypopituitarism is the aim, it is achieved in 83% of the cases.

Analysis of Morbidity and Mortality

The technique described is the result of several modifications which have been introduced throughout ten years in order to obtain a maximal effect on pituitary function with the least morbidity.

Early in our work optic damage occurred in 3 patients. Also, the low degree of hypopituitarism obtained in the initial series of cases made us locate the Yttrium-90 near the floor of the sella and to increase the dose approximately to 20 mC.

In 24 patients in whom this low implant technique was practiced, rhinorrhoea was observed in 8 cases and autopsy findings showed destruction of the bone marrow of the sphenoid and devitalization of the epithelium in the sella turcica and sphenoidal sinus. There were also other signs that the dose used was too high[5]. Due to these findings, we reduced the average implant dose to 15 mC for the normal sized sella. This was divided into 8 or more pellets, localized at least 3 mm below the diaphragm of the sella and 2 mm above its floor.

In 182 patients operated in this way, rhinorrhoea significantly decreased to only 4 cases, but partial visual field defects became evident in 13. The analysis of this change in morbidity was felt to be related to the fact that post-operative radiographic controls showed that the radioactive material—correctly placed in the target point—was mildly displaced, presumably produced by removal of the cannula. In order to avoid this, we first withdraw the cannula to the interclinoidal plane after the implantation of the inactive pellets.

In the last 75 patients in whom this modification was applied, we did not observe visual field defects and rhinorrhoea was present in only 3 of them. This latter complication was present in 15 cases of the total series in 8 of whom it was transient and benign. The remaining 7 developed meningitis, 2 of them dying because they did not seek medical attention. The other 5 improved dramatically with penicillin, rhinorrhoea ceasing after the inflammatory episode with uneventful recovery.

As to other complications, of the 300 patients, 3 of them showed transient oculomotor palsy that disappeared spontaneously after one to three months, in all cases.

Two other patients developed uncontrollable intraoperative haemorrhage and died during surgery. They were diabetic patients in whom hypophysectomy had been indicated for their retinopathy. Post-mortem examinations showed the characteristic diabetic vascular lesions, this being an important contributing factor for the haemorrhage. This complication has not occurred in the remaining 298 cases. Subsequently, we have discontinued and contraindicated the frontal route in patients with diabetic retinopathy.

Diabetes insipidus is frequent in the post-operative period but disappears spontaneously in the majority of the cases. It persists in only 4% and it is readily controlled with pitressin tannate.

Conclusions

According to our experience we conclude that for the intrasellar implantation of radioactive material, the transfrontal route with the technique modifications described is a method worthy of consideration.

The low incidence of complications that are easily controlled, and the fact that this surgical procedure is well tolerated, make this method advisable for obtaining hypopituitarism even in rather poor surgical risk patients.

According to our results diabetic retinopathy is the only contraindication.

References

1. Ferguson, J. D. (1957), Implantation of radioactive material into the pituitary for the control of prostatic cancer. Brit. J. Urol. *29*, 215—221.
2. Forrest, A. P. M., Peebles Brown, D. A. (1955), Pituitary-Radon implant for breast cancer. Lancet *1*, 1054—1055.
3. Frazer, R., Joplin, G. P., Laws, J. W., et al. (1959), Needle implantation of Yttrium seed for pituitary ablation in cases of secondary carcinoma. Lancet *1*, 382—384.
4. Hardy, J. (1971), Transphenoidal hypophysectomy. J. Neurosurg. *34*, 582—594.
5. Jadresic, V. A., Poblete, M., Reid, A., et al. (1965), Therapeutic hypopituitarism induced by stereotaxic transfrontal implantation of Yttrium-90 in patients with breast cancer. J. Clin. Endocr. *25*, 686—697.
6. Molinatti, G. M., Cammanini, R., Massara, F., et al. (1962), Implantation of Yttrium-90 in the sella turcica in cases of acromegaly. J. Clin. Endocr. *22*, 599—611.
7. Poblete, M. (1967), Estudio de la dosis de irradiación intersticial en la hipofisectomía total y parcial mediante el depósito estereotáxico de Y-90 e Ir-192 en la silla turca. Anales del XII Congreso Latinoamericano de Neurocirugía: pp. 853. Lima, Peru.
8. Riechert, T., Mundinger, F. (1959), Stereotaktische Geräte. In: Einführung in die Stereotaktischen Operationen mit einem Atlas des menschlichen Gehirns, Schaltenbrand, G., Bayley, P. Stuttgart: Thieme.
9. — — (1967), Hypophysentumoren, Hypophysektomie. Stuttgart: Thieme.
10. Talairach, J., Szikla, G., Bonis, A., et al. (1962), Destruction stéréotaxique de l'hypophyse non tumorale par les isotopes radioactifs. Presse Med. *70*, 1399—1402; 1449—1451.

Authors' address: M. Poblete, M.D., R. Zamboni, M.D., Department of Stereotactic Neurosurgery, Psychiatric Hospital, Casilla 2677, Santiago, Chile.

Acta Neurochirurgica, Suppl. 21, 165—168 (1974)
© by Springer-Verlag 1974

Department of Neurosurgery, Beth Israel Hospital, Massachusetts General
Hospital and Harvard Medical School, Boston, Mass, U.S.A.

Stereotaxic Thermal Pituitary Ablation

N. T. Zervas and H. Hamlin

During the past seven years we have carried out stereotaxic radiofrequency thermal hypophysectomy in 312 patients. Table 1 lists the
various diseases that were treated by this method.

Table 1. *Thermal Hypophysectomy*

Diabetic Retinopathy	91 cases
Breast Cancer	186 cases
Prostatic Cancer	18 cases
Acromegaly	17 cases

Thermal ablation was produced by introducing an electrode into the
sella turcica using the transnasal transphenoidal route first developed
by Talaraich[1] (1955). Lesions were produced in the pituitary gland by
passing a controlled radiofrequency electrical current through the electrode.
The electrode was designed to permit the projection of a sized stylet at
90° from the electrode tip[2] so as to produce eccentric small heat lesions
in all sectors of the gland. The stylet is composed of soft coiled spring
wire and is very malleable. A bead thermistor is imbedded at the tip to
monitor temperature. It is possible to palpate the margins of the normal
pituitary gland or a pituitary tumor and the diaphragma sellae without
danger of penetrating beyond these structures into adjacent vital areas.
   The advantage of small heat lesions is that they do not extend apparently beyond the confines of the pituitary since heat, once reaching the
diaphragma sellae or the lateral margins of the gland, is carried away by
the flow of either blood in the cavernous sinus and carotid arteries or
cerebrospinal fluid above the diaphragma sellae. This physical barrier to
the transfer of heat beyond the target organ is a protective factor not
inherent in procedures using radioactive substances or deep cold, both
of which can extend beyond the confines of the pituitary gland. To ensure
total hypophysectomy we produce 10–20 small lesions using a tip temperature of 80 °C for 40–60 seconds for each lesion.

Table 2 lists the *visual complications* that have occurred with thermal hypophysectomy. The two transient and one permanent visual impairments that occurred were due to faulty placement of the electrode. In each case the electrode was projected above the diaphragma sellae accidentally. This was due to the use of image amplification in early cases. The definition available with image amplification is not satisfactory for this procedure and it has not been used for many years. Otherwise visual complications have failed to occur despite the fact all operations are now performed under general anesthesia.

Two *operative deaths* occurred, one in 1964 and one in 1966. Both were due to late meningitis occurring many months following operation.

Table 2. *Visual Complications in 312 Patients*

		Permanent	Transient	
Hemianopia		1	2	(5–7 days)
Diplopia		1	2	(3 weeks and 6 weeks)
	Total	2	4	

In each case the diagnosis was not made for several days and the therapy was not instituted in time.

The most troublesome complication of stereotaxic hypophysectomy was *cerebrospinal fluid rhinorrhoea*, which occurred in 15 patients and meningitis which accompanied rhinorrhoea in 5 cases. In all cases the leakage either abated spontaneously or was successfully treated surgically using stereotaxic packing of the sella turcica with fascia lata. The incidence of cerebrospinal fluid rhinorrhoea has been markedly reduced in the past few years and there has only been one case in the last 96 patients. The probability of rhinorrhoea occurring is quite high if steps are not taken to seal the defect in the anterior wall of the sella turcica. Moreover, if increased intracranial pressure is present or if the sella is eroded or destroyed by tumour the incidence of rhinorrhoea will be far greater than normal. Consequently the presence of the latter factors are absolute contraindications for operation as far as the authors are concerned.

The reduction of rhinorrhoea to its present low level of less than 1% was probably due to two factors. The first was packing the electrode track in the pituitary gland with 5–10 small squares of bovine fascia lata*. The packing of the electrode track undoubtedly prevents the

---

* Bovine fascia lata—Ethicon, Inc., Somerville, New Jersey.

passage of cerebrospinal fluid down through the holes in the diaphragma sellae and beyond into the sphenoid sinus. The second tactic we have used for many years is plugging of the bony defect in the anterior wall of the sella turcica with a silicone rubber dowel impregnated with silver. Both manoeuvers together have been extremely effective.

Endocrine data: The best evidence of adequate ablation is the development of hypothyroidism four to eight weeks following operation. 96% of patients did develop hypothyroidism. The most satisfactory early endocrine test for evaluation that was readily available was the I-131 uptake and this ranged from 2–10% in 96% of patients. The determination of human growth hormone level in the serum has been carried out routinely during the past few years only and has been 2 ng/ml or less in 92% of patients.

Breast cancer: We have found that the best candidates for operation are older women with long standing illness dating more than two years from the time of discovery to the time of first metastases or those who have primarily skeletal or cutaneous or pulmonary lesions. A response to oopherectomy or improvement or deterioration following the administration of sex hormones is also a favorable indication. The presence of visceral, liver or brain metastases, while not an absolute contraindication, will seldom be followed by improvement. We operated on 186 patients with metastatic breast carcinoma and 63 demonstrated objective remission and another 41 had a relief from pain for a period of time up to 3 or 6 months. It is interesting to point out that at the recent symposium on breast cancer at Cardiff, Wales[3] strong evidence was presented on the basis of a randomized series comparing hypophysectomy and adrenalectomy that hypophysectomy was superior both as to the incidence of remission and the duration of remission. The results of this study are provocative and should encourage the use of hypophysectomy more often.

In conjuction with Dr. Richard Field and the Retina Foundation in Boston, we have carried out 91 hypophysectomies in patients with *diabetic retinopathy*. Arrest or improvement in visual function was obtained in more than 80% of the patients and is strong evidence that the controversey over the effectiveness of hypophysectomy in diabetic retinopathy should subside. The patients we have selected for hypophysectomy with this complication of diabetes had demonstrable neovascularization of the retina with or without haemorrhage and the pathological process was progressive and threatening vision. Severe deterioration of vision with retinal detachment was a contraindication to operation.

Our most rewarding efforts with thermal ablation have been in the treatment of *acromegaly*. Since the radial stylet can be placed in every sector of the tumour, thermal ablation can be produced around the entire periphery of the tumour as well as the central portions. In such cases, however, we have employed local anaesthesia with an endotracheal tube so as to carefully monitor vision particularly if the diaphragma sellae is elevated. Human growth hormone level in our 17 patients varied from 15 ng/ml to over 400 ng/ml. The average reduction of HGH for the combined series of 17 patients was 91%. This drop was accompanied by almost immediate clinical improvement in most of the patients. Headache subsides and swelling of the hands and feet diminished within the first few days. Glucose intolerance was satisfactorily improved in most patients. Three patients failed to improve satisfactorily. In each case the growth hormone level while falling more than 50% did not come down into the normal range as it did in the remaining patients. These patients had been operated on when our familiarity with the procedure was not great and the electrodes were not placed as optimally as possible. One patient with acromegaly developed transient diplopia. This subsided within three weeks. A second patient developed intrasellar bleeding following operation resulting in chiasmal compression. This was completely reversed following stereotaxic drainage of a large amount of haemorrhagic necrotic material from the tumour cavity.

In conclusion, radiofrequency thermal hypophysectomy is a very low risk procedure and produces satisfactory panhypopituitarism in well over 90% of patients. With careful attention to details any serious or permanent complications can be eliminated.

References

1. Talairach, J. (1955), Appareil de stereotaxie hypophysaire pour voie d'abord nasale. Neurochir. *1*, 127—131.
2. Zervas, N. T. (1969), Stereotaxic radiofrequency surgery of the normal and the abnormal pituitary gland. New Eng. J. Med. *280*, 429—437.
3. Hayward, J. L., Atkins, H. J. B., Falconer, M. A., MacLean, K. S., Salmon, L. F. W., Schurr, P. H., Shaheen, C. H. (1970), Clinical trials comparing transfrontal hypophysectomy with adrenalectomy and with transethmoidal hypophysectomy. Tenovus Workshop, Cardiff, Wales.

Authors' address: N. T. Zervas, M.D., 330 Brookline Avenue, Boston, MA 02215, U.S.A.

Acta Neurochirurgica, Suppl. 21, 169—176 (1974)
© by Springer-Verlag 1974

Neurosurgical University Clinic, Freiburg i. Br., Federal Republic of Germany

Stereotactic Curie-Therapy of Pituitary Adenomas.
A Long-Term Follow-Up Study*

F. Mundinger

With 7 Figures

In the various phases of development of hypophysis surgery the low-risk Curie-therapy has continued to have special clinical relevance. As a primary operative measure the radioactive implant placed intra-tumourally destroys the adenoma or, as a postoperative measure, eliminates the remaining tumour tissue and the hyperfunctioning[16]. We have arrived at this estimation on the basis of comparative examinations of the results produced by operation only, or by Curie-therapy as opposed to conventional radiotherapy, which we have evaluated statistically. The results are presented in a 1967 monograph[12], as well as in other publications[7, 8, 9, 10, 11].

Microsurgery doubtlessly presents a further surgical aid in permitting operations to be undertaken using a transsphenoid approach, as Schloffer[15] had demonstrated as early as 1907, or an endonasal approach, as Hirsch[6] had employed in 1910, and which was further developed by Halstead[5] (1910) and Cushing[3] (1912). Yet microsurgery has not solved all the problems, as may sometimes appear, neither in view of complications or recidives, nor for the combination of transcranial and transsphenoidal approaches, as used by Burian[2]. In passing, let it be mentioned that the transcranial approach was first registered as being used by Fedor Krause in 1905 and shortly thereafter was further elaborated by Frazier (1913), Dandy et al.[4]. We must nevertheless await the comparative results of long-term postoperative observation before evaluating the advantages of microsurgery on the hypophysis.

* Supported by Special Research Grant, Gehirnforschung und Sinnes-physiologie (S F B 70, III d), of the Deutsche Forschungsgemeinschaft.

However, we can today present an evaluation of stereotactic Curie-
therapy on the basis of long-term results dating from 1953[14].

Results

We performed 288 pituitary operations from a total of 487 Curie-
therapy treatments. Despite our efforts, it was unfortunately impossible
for us to obtain objective postoperative results and catamnesia from
all patients.

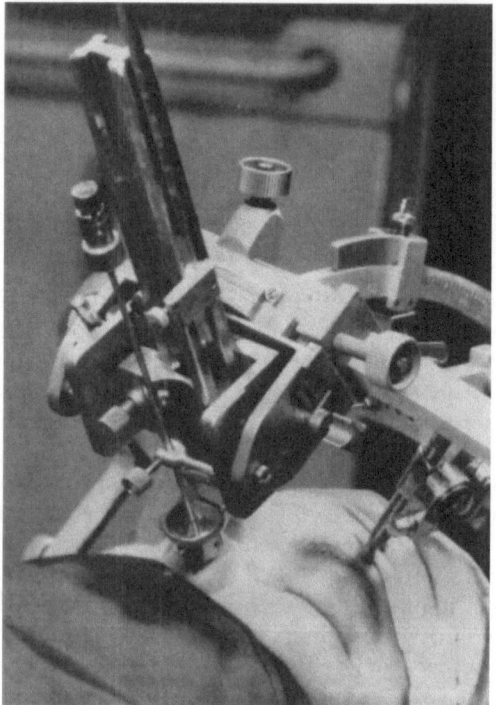

Fig. 1

We did succeed in obtaining data for 152 patients, working partly
in co-operation with Bräun. We examined a first series of 79 patients
who had been implanted with gold-198-graphite seeds between 1953
and 1961 using a transfrontal approach. The first patients in this series
also received phosphorus-32 implants. The median postoperative observation time was 10.9 ± 2.1 years. Then we have by contrast a second
series of 73 patients operated on between 1962–1968 using mostly a
transsphenoid approach and implanted for the most part with
iridium-192 and the rest with iridium-192 combined with yttrium-90.
Median postoperative observation time is 4.0 ± 1.8 years for this series.

Method

After calculating the intrasellar target co-ordinates and the adjustment parameter we bore a path into the sphenoid cavity using the bore and guidance tubule and inject a filling composed of an fibrogenous solution. Subsequently the anterior sellar wall is perforated with a hand drill and the implantation probe, which has a diameter of 1.3 mm, is

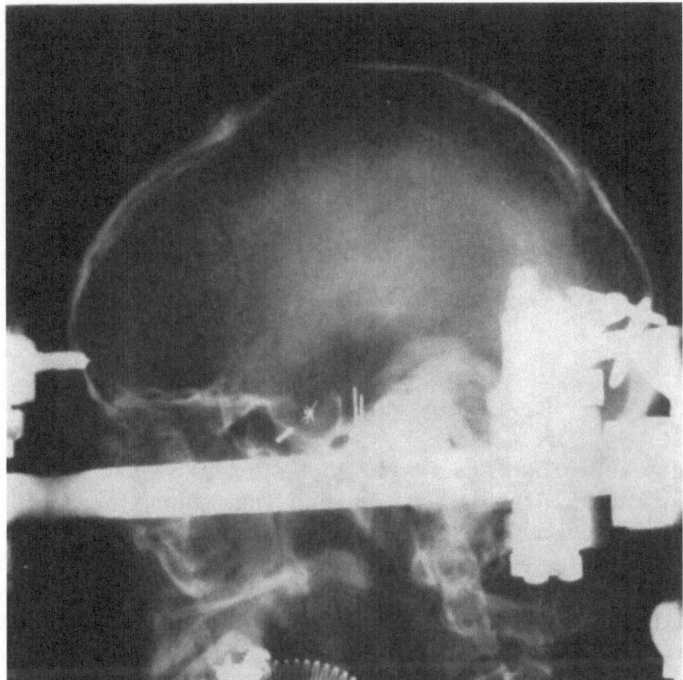

Fig. 2

moved towards its target (Fig. 1). Once we have made certain that there is no cyst or extensive subdiaphragmal cistern in the basal region, we implant the radioactive seed. Finally we close the opening of the perforation in the anterior sellar wall with a gold-nickel screw 1.4 mm in diameter (Fig. 2). We now carry out the entire stereotactic procedure including dosimetry using a computer programme. Modification of the target apparatus and development of computer programmes have been carried out in collaboration with Birg.

No operative mortality, overall mortality 15.5%. 4 patients (2.9%) died in the clinic or later as a result of the operation and four others

(2.9%) from recidives. Of the patients with eosinophile adenomas 89% survived up to 8 years after the operation and 79% of the chromophobe adenoma patients have survival times ranging up to 16 years subsequent to operation. The follow-up mortality lies at 21% for the patients in series I, 7.8% for series II. According to an early evaluation made in 1967, 54% of those solely operated on for chromophobe adenomas were still alive 8 years after the implant. In comparison, Bakay 1950[1] gives the figures of 56% surviving up to 18 years in the Olivecrona series and Tönnis, Oberdisse, and Weber 1953[17] state that 29% were still alive

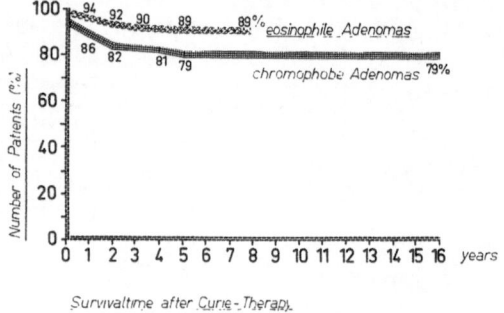

Fig. 3. Survivaltime after Curie-therapy

after 4 years in the Tönnis series, but after 10 years this figure was reduced to 3.6%. Our survival rates are thus notably higher.

Vision diminished for only 14% of the chromophobe adenomas in series I and 14% were already blind prior to the operation (Fig. 4). In series II vision worsened for 9%. However, in series II with iridium 50% of the patients showed visual improvement, compared to only 31% for series I. There were no recidives noted for a total of 86% of the series I patients and 91% of the patients in series II.

Even more impressive are the long-term results for the visual fields (Fig. 5). From series II 75% of the patients implanted with iridium-192 improved due to a reduction in pressure on the chiasma; only in 3% did the condition worsen. Taken together, 84% of series I patients and 97% of those in series II showed no progression of symptoms or recidives.

In diagram 6 the evaluation of the vision acuity and visual fields of eosinophile adenomas may be seen. The inner circle represents series I, the outer series II. Here especially we note the improved functional effect of iridium-192 treatment. Vision worsened for 16% in series I —marked in dark grey—and in series II for only 10%, whereas 24% of those in series II improved—note the light grey. On the right it can be seen that no cases showed a decline in visual fields. At 35% series II

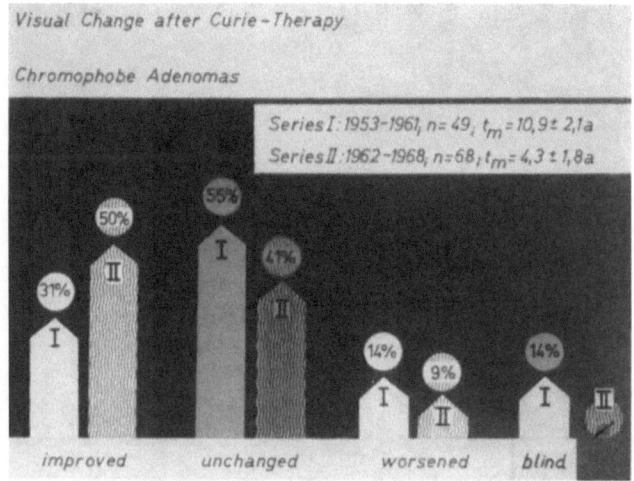

Fig. 4. Visual change after Curie-therapy. Chromophobe adenomas

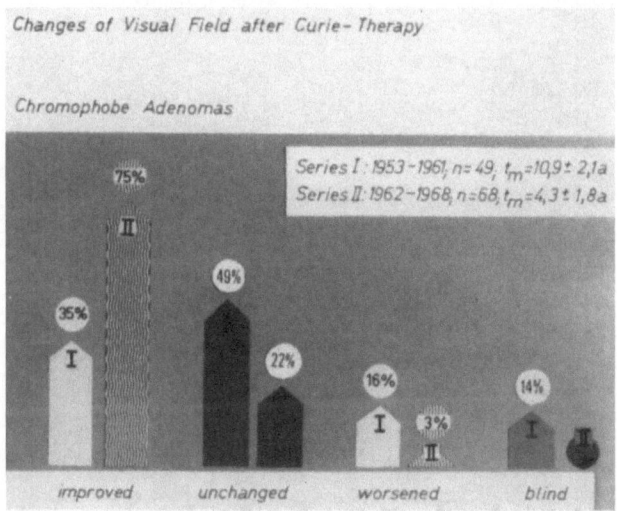

Fig. 5. Changes of visual field after Curie-therapy. Chromophobe adenomas

shows a higher percentage of improved cases—recorded in light grey. Acromegalic changes declined in 36% for series I and 64%—or twice the figure for series I—for series II, while increasing for only 9% in each of the two series. The determination of the growth hormone has also objectively confirmed these results. Characteristic of the functional effect of iridium-192 is its ability to normalise the raised STH values leaving the other adenotrope systems for the most part untouched.

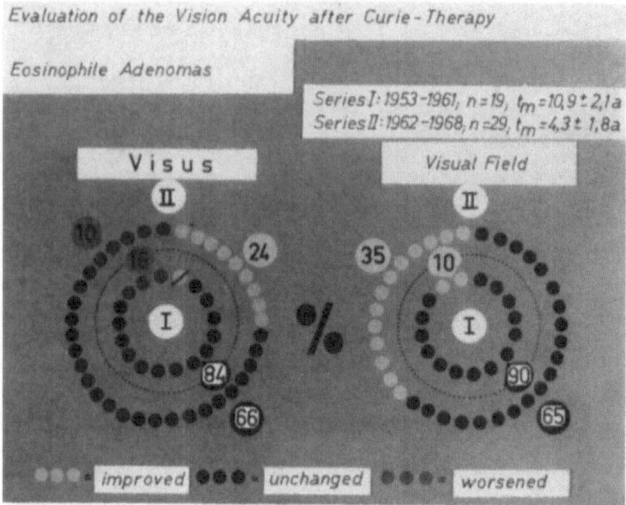

Fig. 6. Evaluation of the vision acuity after Curie-therapy. Eosinophile adenomas

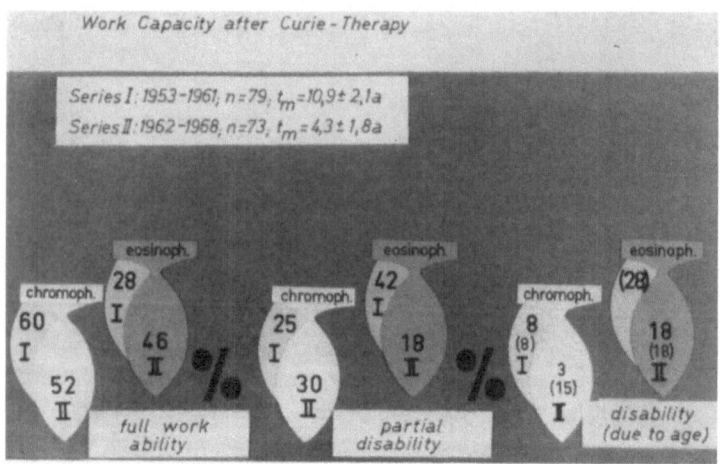

Fig. 7. Work capacity after Curie-therapy

In conclusion let us consider the patients' work capacity, the steepest of all criteria since it involves both objective and subjective symptoms of illness (Fig. 7). 8% of series I chromophobe adenoma patients are characterized as unable to work, and a further 8%, figures in parentheses, could no longer work due to age. Only 3% of the patients treated in series II could no longer work due to illness. It is of course natural to find that for the patients with eosinophilic adenomas, which engender endocrinal changes, there was a higher percentage of work disability. However, our figures here correlate with those given in 1967 by Olive-crona for open operations, as do the other data as well. Total work ability occurs in circa ½ of our cases and partial disability for ⅓.

Summary

The long-term results of postoperative observation for up to 18 years, as presented here, confirm our earlier statement:

1. Compared to conventional operational methods the primary intra-sellar stereotactic Curie-therapy is at least as effective as or provides an effective complement to the former when employed as secondary postoperative irradiation treatment. There are no similar long-term observational results for microsurgery at present to permit a comparison.

2. Curie-therapy is characterized by a modest operational taxing of the patient and a low rate of operational risk.

3. Functionally speaking, iridium-192 is more effective than gold-198 and yttrium-90.

4. Following both primary and secondary implantations, the Curie-therapy improves the recidive rate considerably and reduces it to very low percentages.

5. The survival times are lengthened to a decisive degree in comparison to other methods of treatment.

References

1. Bakay, L. (1950), The results of 300 pituitary adenoma operations. J. Neurosurg. *7*, 240—255.
2. Burian, K. (1970), Mikrochirurgie der Hypophyse. Jahrestagung der Deutschen Gesellschaft für Neurochirurgie, Göttingen. In: Fortschritte auf dem Gebiet der Neurochirurgie, hrsg. von K.-H. Bushe. Stuttgart: Hippokrates-Verlag.
3. Cushing, H. (1912), The pituitary body and its disorders. Philadelphia-London: Lippincott.
4. Dandy, W. E. (1933), Benign tumors in the third ventricle of the brain. Springfield, Ill.: Ch. C Thomas.
5. Halstead, A. E. (1910), Remarks on the operative treatment of tumors of the hypophysis. Report of two cases operated on by an oronasal method. Surg. Gynec. Obstet. *10*, 494—502.
6. Hirsch, O. (1910), Endonasal method of removal of hypophyseal tumors. With report of two successfull cases. J. Amer. med. Ass. *55*, 772—774.
7. Mundinger, F. (1961), Langzeitergebnisse der stereotaktischen Radio-Isotopen-Bestrahlung von Hypophysentumoren (im Vergleich zur trans-kraniellen offenen Operation). Strahlenther. *116*, 523—535.
8. — (1963), Die interstitielle Radio-Isotopen-Bestrahlung von Hirn-tumoren mit vergleichenden Langzeitergebnissen zur Röntgentiefen-therapie. Acta neurochir. *9*, 89—109.

9. Mundinger, F. (1969), Die intraselläre protrahierte Langzeitbestrahlung von Hypophysenadenomen mittels stereotaktischer Implantation von Iridium[192]. Acta Radiol. (Scand). *8*, 55—62.
10. — (1969), Techniques and indications for the interstitial irradiation of brain and pituitary tumours with radionuclides. Kerntechnik, Isotopentechnik und -Chemie *11*, 333—345.
11. — (1970), Brain tumour therapy by interstitial application of radioactive isotopes. Monograph: Radionuclide applications in neurology and neurosurgery, ed. by Paoletti, P., and Yen Wang. Springfield, Ill.: Ch. C Thomas.
12. — Radiohypophysectomy. Progr. Neurol. Surg. Basel-New York: F. Karger. Im Druck.
13. — Riechert, T. (1967), Hypophysentumoren — Hypophysektomie. Stuttgart: G. Thieme.
14. Riechert, T., Mundinger, F. (1959), Stereotaktische Geräte. In: Einführung in die stereotaktischen Operationen mit einem Atlas des menschlichen Gehirns. Schaltenbrand, G., Bailey, P. Stuttgart: G. Thieme.
15. Schloffer, H. (1907), Erfolgreiche Operation eines Hypophysentumors auf nasalem Wege. Wien. klin. Wschr. *20*, 621—624.
16. Talairach, J., Bonis, A., Szikla, G., Schaub, G., Bancaud, J., Covello, L., Bordas-Ferrer, M. (1970), Stereotaxic implantation of radioactive isotopes in functional pituitary surgery: Technique and results. In: Radionuclide applications in neurology and neurosurgery, ed. by Yen Wang and P. Paoletti. Springfield, Ill.: Ch. C Thomas.
17. Tönnis, W., Oberdisse, K., Weber, E. (1953), Bericht über 264 operierte Hypophysenadenome. Acta neurochir. *3*, 113—130.

Author's address: Prof. F. Mundinger, Neurosurgical Clinic, University of Freiburg, Hugstetterstraße 55, D-7800 Freiburg i. Br., Federal Republic of Germany.

Acta Neurochirurgica, Suppl. 21, 177—183 (1974)
© by Springer-Verlag 1974

Department of Neurosurgery, Karolinska Sjukhuset, Stockholm 60, Sweden

Stereotaxic Treatment of Craniopharyngiomas

E.-O. Backlund

With 4 Figures

The modern adjuncts of improved anaesthesia, endocrine supervision and therapy and also of microsurgery have reduced the risks confined to radical surgery in craniopharyngiomas. Nevertheless, the overall operative mortality reported in recent papers approximates 15%. In addition, many of the survivors are reported as more or less disabled. Against this background the need for improved methods of treatment is obvious. By means of stereotaxis these lesions can be punctured for biopsies, decompression of cysts and intracavitary radionuclide treatment.

The first case treated according to these principles was reported by Leksell and Lidén in 1952. Since then, occasional cases and small series treated by similar techniques have been reported by other authors (Klar 1953, Wycis et al. 1954, Northfield 1957, Riechert and Mundinger 1957, Campbell and Hudson 1960, Hankinson 1961, Overton and Sheffel 1963, Volkov et al. 1963, Bond et al. 1965, Badmaev et al. 1969, Trippi et al. 1969, Nakayama et al. 1971). In many of these the results were difficult to estimate and, in addition, on five occasions the outcome was fatal. This made some of the authors doubtful concerning the value of their tentative efforts. Some, however, were not entirely discouraged by the results and advocated this type of treatment at least in recurrent or desperate cases. Apparently, the results were not convincing enough to make this policy generally accepted. It was necessary to develop the method systematically and to compare the results of this mode of treatment in consecutive patients with those generally obtained by conventional surgery.

At the Department of Neurosurgery at Karolinska sjukhuset, Stockholm, a treatment programme for these lesions has been worked out and since 1966 applied to all craniopharyngioma cases (Leksell et al. 1967, Backlund 1969, Backlund et al. 1972).

Methods

Primarily rounded portions of the suspected cystic tumour are chosen
for puncture. Before incision of the dura, the anatomy of the proposed
puncture track is studied with stereotaxically directed transdural echo-
encephalography (Backlund and Levander 1970) and in some cases
with angiography (Fig. 1). The volumes of cysts found at the puncture
are calculated by means of a radioactivity dilution method and their
configurations are studied by the injection of a little amount of air.
If no cyst is found at the puncture, an attempt to obtain a biopsy is
made. For the cyst treatment, the radionuclide chosen is ^{90}Y in a
colloidal preparation obtained from the Radiochemical Centre,
Amersham. For the sake of accurate dosimetry, variations of the volume
and the form of the cyst should be avoided during the operation. Equal
amounts of cyst fluid and yttrium solution are thus aspirated and
injected, respectively. The activity to be injected is determined by a
radiation dose formula based on the beta-dose calculations derived by
Loevinger et al. (1956). During the first postoperative days the distribution of the isotope in the body is studied. The "Bremsstrahlung"
from the ^{90}Y is sufficient to obtain scintigrams of the distribution
within the head. This examination is performed routinely as well as
measurements of samples from the blood and CSF compartments.
As more than 95% of the radiation dose is delivered within the first
five half-lives, decompression of the cyst can well be carried out about
two weeks after the radionuclide injection, if required. After such an
evacuation a contrast medium can be injected into the cyst to outline
its anatomy and this is of great value during the follow-up. Useful
compounds are the aqueous suspensions of barium sulphate in a micro-
crystalline form or tantalum powder.

For the treatment of solid tumour parts verified at the diagnostic
puncture, the gamma unit described by Leksell (1968, 1971) and Larsson
et al. (1970) is used (Fig. 2). The procedure is performed by cross firing
of the target region by 179 narrow beams of ^{60}Co gamma radiation distributed within a spherical sector. The beams are radially directed towards the centre of this sector, in which the predetermined tumour
target point is positioned. The apparatus was primarily developed
for functional radiosurgery. Because of this, the system of apertures for
each individual beam and the spatial distribution of the ^{60}Co sources
were designed to give disc-shaped dose distributions with very steep
dose gradients in the border zones of the lesions to be produced. For
the treatment of solid craniopharyngiomas such a dose distribution may
be too small to be optimal. To avoid this obstacle, and in order to adapt
the irradiated volume to the shape of the tumour, a number of target
points in a predetermined spatial pattern are used).

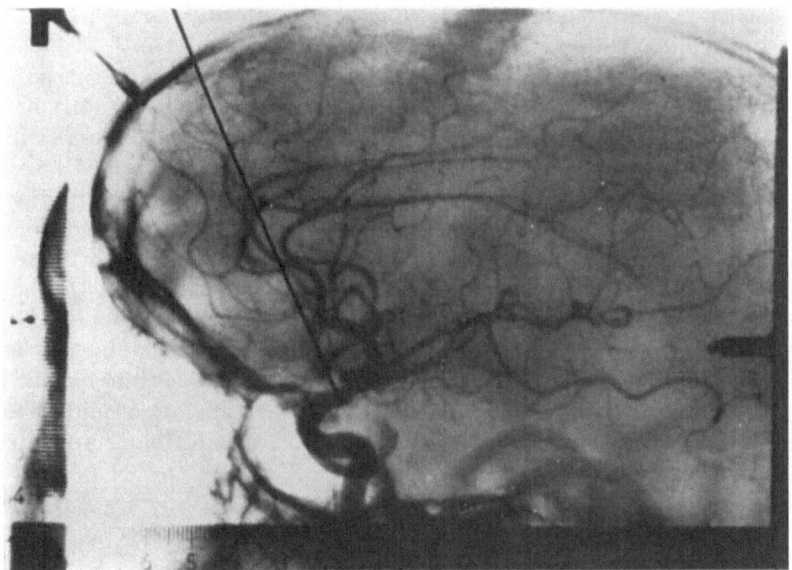

Fig. 1

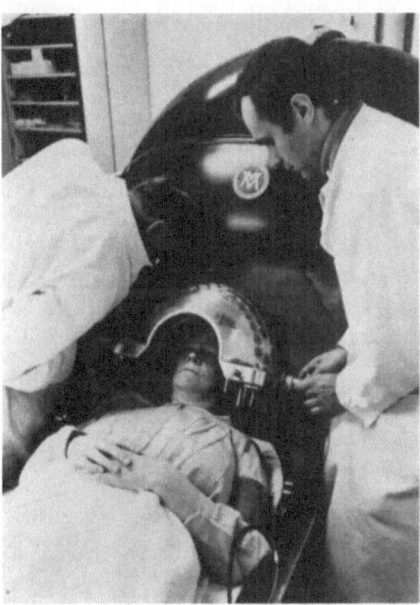

Fig. 2

The operative procedure is started with the application to the patients head of a special circular fixation frame. Under local anaesthesia, it is secured by four steel pins to the outer table of the skull. The purpose of this frame is to obtain accurate fixation of the patient in the irradiation unit. The coordinate frame is then fixed to the circular frame and the routine procedure for coordinate determination is performed. The target point or points are chosen in the central region of the solid portion of the tumour and at a safe distance from the optic pathways and from the hypothalamus. At sites determined by the X and Y coordinates burr holes are made in plexiglass sheets in the side of the circular frame. The fixation axes of the collimator helmet are inserted into the burr holes with an adjustment along the transverse axis according to the Z determination (Fig. 2). The movable operating table with the collimator helmet is then moved into position in the irradiation unit. The irradiation time required for the delivery of 5 krads to the centre of a human head is about half an hour.

Material

Our material from the years 1966 to 1969 has recently been analysed (Backlund 1972a and b) and consists of 14 consecutive cases. Three cases were recurrences after major surgery. In one case only, the tumour was found to be without cystic portions. Radio-yttrium was injected into the cysts, the total number of which were 17. The dose to the cyst wall was 20 krads. During the observation time (average 2.5 years) X-rays showed a gradual decrease of the size of the cysts (Fig. 3). Clinical improvement—even in pituitary function—appeared in the majority of cases. With the exception of one unilateral blindness of obscure origin, no complications were encountered. The immediate postoperative course of all cases was very smooth. It has to be compared with the often dramatic postoperative periods following conventional surgical attempts at craniopharyngioma removal.

The occupations of the patients at the end of the follow-up were as follows:

Attending school or university	5 cases
Housewife	2 cases
Factory worker	2 cases
Carpenter	1 case
Nurse	1 case
Office clerk	1 case
Disabled by postoperative epilepsy after transfrontal operation	1 case
Not working—under treatment	1 case

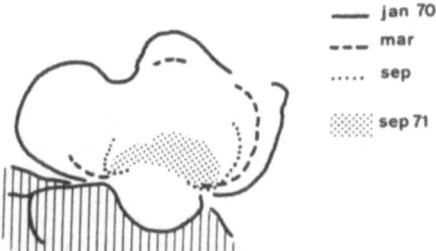

——— jan 70

--- mar

..... sep

▓▓ sep 71

Fig. 3. M. B. 35 years. Compound sketch from consecutive X-rays after yttrium administration. A continuous and gradual decrease of the cyst size is shown

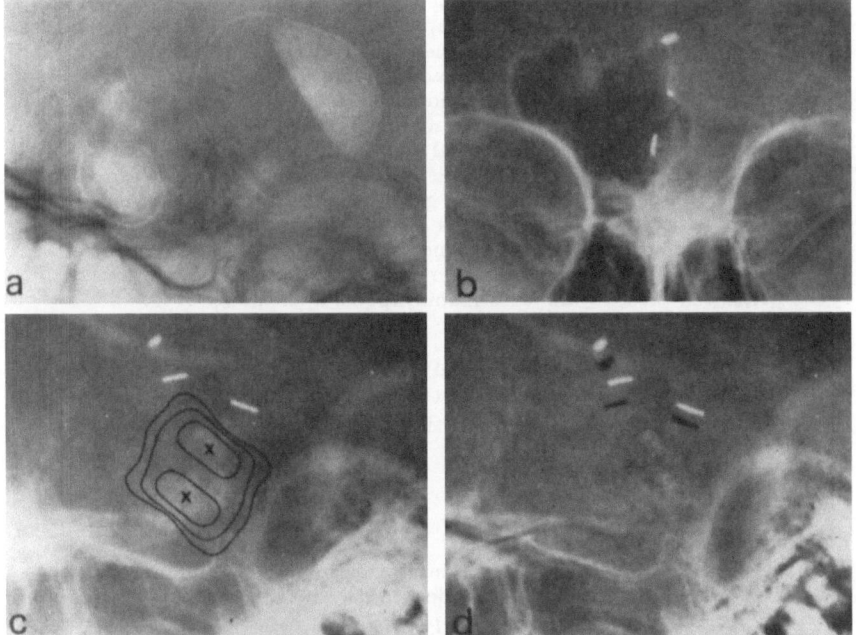

Fig. 4. N. J. 15 years. Previous to the radiosurgery, there cysts were treated with yttrium-90, two of them are outlined in (a). After the cyst collapse, indicators were inserted after biopsy at the top of the residual solid tumour (b and c). The two target points (x, x) for the radiosurgical procedure are indicated in (c) as well as the isodose diagram for the summated dose distribution used in this case. The 10, 20 and 50% isodose curves are out-lined. With the use of the subtraction technique, stereotaxic X-rays from the radiosurgical procedure (white indicators) and 8 months later (black indicators) are compared in (d). The tumour shrinkage is indicated by the different locations of the indicators

The results indicate that yttrium administration is always advocated as the treatment for expansive cysts, which are most often responsible for the clinical problems in cases of craniopharyngioma.

Finally, a brief description is given of 4 cases, treated in the gamma unit. In one case, with an entirely solid tumour, this was the primary treatment. The remaining 3 had residual solid tumour portions after the cyst treatment. To the centre of the area chosen for irradiation a single dose of 5000 rads was delivered. Its margins received at least 300 rads. The first case has been observed for 3.5 years without displaying any deterioration, although her only symptom, secondary amenorrhoea, did not improve. The second case followed a very satisfactory course. Of the main initial symptoms, the visual disturbances disappeared and the diabetes insipidus was ameliorated after the cyst treatment with yttrium-90, whereas the secondary amenorrhoea remained unimproved. As the solid portion of the tumour was almost filling up the whole sella, the position of the pituitary gland could not be imagined when the solid tumour portion was to be treated and the secreting parenchyma of the compressed anterior lobe may well have received a considerable radiation dose. This possibility is supported by the decrease in cortisol and PBI values after the irradiation. Later on, these values became normal and the pituitary apparently recovered as the patient began to menstruate spontaneously, became pregnant and gave birth to a normal child. The growth of the tumour, was apparently arrested by the treatment. In the remaining two patients the observation period is too short to allow any conclusions concerning the clinical effect. The treatment however, appeared to cause arrest of tumour growth within the irradiated area, in one case manifested as a shrinkage (Fig. 4).

The results indicate that it is possible without surgical risks, to treat by stereotaxic radiosurgery selected portions of craniopharyngiomas and apparently, to obtain obliteration of the areas irradiated.

References

1. Backlund, E. O. (1969), Stereotaxic treatment of craniopharyngiomas. In Nobel Symposium 10: Disorders of the skull base region (Eds. Hamberger, C. A., Wersäll, J.), pp. 237—244. Stockholm: Almqvist & Wiksell.
2. — Levander, B. (1970), Echoencephalographic sounding of the puncture track in stereotaxic brain tumour biopsy. Acta Neurol. Scand. 46, 529.
3. — (1972a), Studies on craniopharyngiomas. III. Stereotaxic treatment with intracystic yttrium-90. Acta Chir. Scand. 139, 237—247.
4. — (1972b), Studies on craniopharyngiomas. IV. Stereotaxic treatment with radiosurgery. Acta Chir. Scand. 139, 344—351.
5. — Johansson, L., Sarby, B. (1972), Studies on craniopharyngiomas. II. Treatment by stereotaxis and radiosurgery. Acta Chir. Scand. 138, 749—759.

6. Badmaev, K. N., Balalamutova, H. P., Vaknovetsky, B. P. (1969), On the problem of neurosurgical treatment of patients with cranio-pharyngiomas. Vop. Neirokhir. *33*, 13—16.
7. Bond, W. H., Richards, D., Turner, E. (1965), Experiences with radio-active gold in the treatment of craniopharyngioma. J. Neurol. Neuro-surg. Psychiat. *28*, 30—39.
8. Campbell, J. B., Hudson, F. M. (1960), Craniobuccal origin, signs and treatment of craniopharyngiomas. Surg. Gynecol. Obstet. *III*, 183—191.
9. Hankinson, J. (1961), Discussion contribution (2nd Int. Congr. Neurol. Surg.). Excerpta Med. Int. Congr. Ser. *36*, E 7.
10. Klar, E. (1953), Zur gezielten Punktionsbehandlung bestimmter Hirn-tumoren. Langenbecks Arch. Chir. *276*, 117—121.
11. Larsson, B., Lidén, K., Sarby, B. (1970), Techniques for irradiation of small intracranial structures through the intact skull. Proc. 9th Symposium Neuroradiologicum.
12. Leksell, L., Lidén, K. (1952), A therapeutic trial with radioactive isotopes in cystic brain tumour. Radioisotope techniques I, Med. and physiol. appl. 1—4.
13. — Backlund, E. O., Johansson, L. (1967), Treatment of craniopharyn-giomas. Acta Chir. Scand. *133*, 345—350.
14. — (1968), Cerebral radiosurgery I. Grammathalamotomy in two cases of intractable pain. Acta Chir. Scand. *134*, 585—595.
15. — (1971), Stereotaxis and radiosurgery. An operative system. Spring-field, Ill.: Ch. C Thomas.
16. Loevinger, R., Japha, E. M., Brownell, G. L. (1956), In radiation dosi-metry (Eds. Hine & Brownell). New York: Academic Press.
17. Nakayama, T., Kodama, T., Matsukado, Y. (1971), Treatment of inoperable craniopharyngioma, with special reference to the injection of [198]Au into the cystic cavity. Brain Nerve (Tokyo) *23*, 509—513.
18. Northfield, D. W. C. (1957), Rathke-pouch tumours. Brain *80*, 293—312.
19. Overton, M. C., Sheffel, D. D. (1963), Recurrent cystic formation in craniopharyngioma treated with radioactive chromic phosphate. J. Neurosurg. *20*, 707—710.
20. Riechert, T., Mundinger, F. (1957), Erfahrungen der stereotaktischen Hypophysenoperationen mit Radioisotopen. Chirurg *28*, 145—151.
21. Trippi, A. C., Garner, J. T., Kassabian, J. T., et al. (1969), A new ap-proach to inoperable craniopharyngiomas. Amer. J. Surg. *118*, 307—310.
22. Volkov, A. A., Vaskin, I. S., Zobina, M. M., Muratkhodzhaev, N. (1963), The use of colloidal radioactive isotopes for radiotherapy of cranio-pharyngiomas. Med. Radiol. (Moskva) *8*, 23—29.
23. Wycis, H. T., Robbins, R., Spiegel-Adolf, M., Meszaros, J., Spiegel, E. A. (1954), Treatment of a cystic craniopharyngioma by injection of radioactive P[32]. Confin. Neurol. *14*, 193—202.

Author's address: Dr. E.-O. Backlund, Department of Neurosurgery, Karolinska Sjukhuset, Stockholm 60, Sweden.

Acta Neurochirurgica, Suppl. 21, 185—191 (1974)
© by Springer-Verlag 1974

Departamento de Neurocirugia Ciudad Sanitaria "Virgen del Rocio",
Sevilla, Spain

Stereotactic Hypothalamotomy in Erethic Children

V. E. Arjona

It is possible to control aggressive behaviour by surgical means. A fair number of operations, mainly stereotactic, have been reported aiming to produce lesions in structures related to emotional pathways and a high rate of success has been claimed by several authors. These operations include frontal leucotomy (Freeman and Watts 1950), lesions in the orbital cortex (Scoville 1951, Knight 1964), dorsomedian thalamotomy (Spiegel et al. 1949), amygdalotomy (Narabayashi 1961, Narabayashi et al. 1963, Heimburger et al. 1966, Vaernet and Madsen 1970), cingulectomy (Lebeau 1952, Lebeau 1954, Sano 1954, Ballantine et al. 1967), anterior thalamotomy (Spiegel and Wycis 1953, Handa et al. 1961), fornicotomy (Sano 1957) etc.

Some of these operations have also been done in our department and in particular with amygdalotomy and anterior thalamotomy, good relief was attained in a variety of aggressive states of diverse aetiology. Nevertheless there has been a group of patients in whom all the above mentioned operations have consistently failed. I am referring to the so-called oligophrenia erethica or agitated idiocy. These are children with low IQ and a wild form of aggressiviness who live in constant agitation, destroying everything they can get hold of. They are auto-aggressive as well as hetero-aggressive, presenting a constant danger to other children. Four of the patients came to hospital with multiple swellings and haematomas due to injuries they had themselves inflicted. They do not respond to medical therapy and as they grow older their erethism becomes more marked.

Following experimental work by Bard (1939), Hess (1947, 1949), Beattie et al. (1930, 1932), Ingram et al. (1951, 1952), Kurotsu (1954) and others who provided evidence that the hypothalamus plays an important role in the emotional circuit and the clinico-physiological work of Sano et al. (1962, 1966, 1970) who obtained good results with lesions in the posteromedial hypothalamus in a wide variety of aggressive states, we decided to produce stereotactic lesions in the hypothalamus of erethic children having failed previously with all other forms of treatment.

Analysis of Clinical Material

From July 1970 to May 1972, eleven patients had postero-medial hypothalamotomy. Bilateral lesions were performed in ten patients; in the remaining case a unilateral lesion only was done. Seven were males and four females and their ages ranged from 3 to 13 years.

The clinical picture was similar in all patients and all had erethism to a marked degree. Four patients were also epileptic, three had Grand Mal attacks and one Petit Mal. One had a spastic paraparesis. Three patients had a previous history of encephalitis in early childhood and two were born cyanotic after prolonged labour.

The EEG showed non-specific abnormalities in four cases. It was normal in three while in the four patients having epilepsy a wide range of abnormalities in accordance with this disease was observed. All patients were seen by a psychiatrist before they came to surgery and in most of them the IQ could not be tested due to their agitation and lack of cooperation. It was thought they were all well below 80.

Air-encephalography was also done in all cases in order to exclude the existence of a space occupying lesion and to determine the degree of ventricular dilatation. Six patients had a marked degree of cerebral atrophy with big ventricles and large amounts of air over the convexity. In the remaining five patients the air-encephalography was normal.

Two patients had previous operations for their aggressive behaviour. One had bilateral stereotactic amygdalotomy and dorsomedian thalamotomy. The second one had, in addition to these, bilateral lesions in the anterior nuclei of the thalamus. Their erethism did not improve after the operations but they did not have any demonstrable side-effects either.

The operation was always done under general anesthesia. Each side was operated on a different session with about 10 to 12 days interval. Leksell stereotactic apparatus (Leksell 1949, 1971) was used and the ventricles were outlined by ventriculography through a frontal burr-hole. The lesions were made with the Cooper cryogenic system (Cooper et al. 1962, 1963). The temperature at the cannula tip was dropped to $-60°$ being maintained at $0°$, $-20°$, and $-40°$ for a period of one minute each. A final lesion at $-60°$ for 90 seconds was made.

The lesions were centered 3 mm below the mid-point of the inter-

Table 1

No.	Sex	Age	Previous Diseases	Clinical Picture	Previous Operations	Complications	Results	Follow-up (Months)
1	F	7	prolonged labour	violent behaviour mental retardation	MD. NA. amygdala	—	no aggressions	25
2	M	7	—	aggressive behaviour mental retardation	—	—	no aggressions	17
3	F	8	—	violent behaviour mental retardation epilepsy	—	—	no aggressions fits improved	17
4	M	6	mother had germ. measles d. preg.	aggressive behaviour mental retardation	—	dystonic mov. upper limbs	no aggressions	17
5	M	13	—	aggressive behaviour mental retardation epilepsy	—	—	no aggressions epilepsy impved.	8
6	M	13	prolonged labour	violent behaviour mental retardation spastic paraparesis	—	hyperthermia increase spasticity	no aggressions	8
7	F	11	encephalitis	aggressive behaviour mental retardation	MD. amygdala	—	no aggressions	7
8	M	6	encephalitis	aggressive behaviour mental retardation	—	—	no aggressions	6
9	M	3	—	aggressive behaviour mental retardation epilepsy	—	—	no aggressions epilepsy impved.	4
10	M	9	encephalitis	aggressive behaviour mental retardation	—	—	improved	4
11	F	5	—	aggressive behaviour mental retardation	—	—	no aggressions	3

commisural line (CA–CP) and 3 to 4 mm lateral to the wall of the third ventricle. The estimated size of the lesion was 5 mm diameter. During operation blood pressure, pulse rate, respiration and pupillary size were carefully observed. It was a common finding that the pupils became smaller as the lesion was started, then became larger as the lesion was about to be completed, regaining miosis again when the temperature returned to $+37°$. Nevertheless pupillary changes were not consistent and in any case are of doubtful value in patients under general anesthesia. A fall in blood pressure and slowing of the pulse was observed in almost every patient, which persisted for several weeks. Changes in respiration or alterations in ocular movements were not found.

After operation the patients remained hypothermic for 12 to 24 hours and after that period they had hyperthermia which usually lasted for two or three days, settling down thereafter. During the first postoperative hours they were also extremely agitated having to be sedated for 24 hours.

Results

All patients improved after operation. In all the auto- and hetero-aggression disappeared. Agitation also improved enormously and they were able to live at home and mix with other children. Four patients have been able to attend special schools where they appear to be making progress. Two others now go to their village school. Their families think they have become more intelligent after the operation but this may be due to the loss of their aggressive behaviour.

Two patients get excited at times and on the whole they are more excitable than a normal child. The remaining five patients are reported by their families to be as quiet or even quieter that their brothers and sisters.

Of the four patients who had epilepsy, all had fits after the operation but their number has been reduced and they appear to be more easily controlled with drugs.

Complications

Serious complications occurred in two patients. The first one developed hyperthermia of central origin after the second lesion was made. It persisted for two months and then slowly disappeared. He had a spastic paraparesis and the spasticity increased after the operation.

Another patient immediatley after operation developed dystonic movements in both upper limbs, which persisted during the month he was in hospital. When he was seen a month later in the follow-up clinic the movements had completely cleared-up.

Discussion

The zone of the hypothalamus where the lesions have been made includes the posterior portion of the posterior hypothalamic nucleus and the dorsal longitudinal fasciculus and corresponds to zone b of Kurotsu (1954). It is the zone which some authors (Sano 1970, Schvarcz et al. 1972) have found in man to respond to stimulation with signs of sympathetic discharge. The lesions should be large enough to destroy most of this zone and sufficiently small not to interfere with the lateral hypothalamus. The size should be kept under 6 mm diameter as large lesions in this area are reported to produce stupor and anorexia in animals (Sano 1966).

From the present study and from the series already published it seems that the operation is quite safe if the lesions are accurately placed. It is possible that the persistent hyperthermia which one of the patients presented during the first two months after operation could be due to involvement of the zone c of Kurotsu in the lateral hypothalamus which he found to play an important role in temperature regulation. The cause of the dystonic picture that another patient presented remains obscure.

Stereotactic hypothalamotomy has been in our experience the only procedure that has brought persistent relief to this type of erethic children. It is possible that this operation should be extended to other types of violent behaviour. It is our impression that lesions to be effective should be bilateral. Nevertheless it is possible that in milder forms of aggressive behaviour improvement might be obtained with a unilateral lesion. One of the cases of the present series improved so much after the first lesion that it was thought wise to postpone the second lesion until signs of recurrence appear. Although the follow-up is still short this patient continues calmed.

References

1. Ballantine, H. T., Cassidy, W. L., Flanigan, N. B., Marino, R. (1967), Stereotaxic anterior cingulotomy for neuropsychiatric illness and intractable pain. J. Neurosurg. *26*, 488—495.
2. Bard, P. (1939), Central nervous mechanisms for emotional behaviour patterns on animals. Research Publications, Association for Research in Nervous and Mental Disease *19*, 190—218.
3. Beattie, J. (1932), Hypothalamic mechanisms. Canad. med. Ass. J. *26*, 400—405.
4. — Brow, C. R., Long, C. N. H. (1930), Physiological and anatomical evidence for the existence of nerve tracts connecting the hypothalamus with spinal sympathetic centres. Proc. Roy. Soc. *106*, 253—275.
5. Cooper, I. S., Grissman, F., Johnston, R. (1962), A complete system for cryogenic surgery. St. Barnabas Hosp. Med. Bull. *1*, 11—19.

6. Cooper, I. S. (1963), Cryogenic Surgery. New Eng. J. Med. *268*, 743—756.
7. Freeman, W., Watts, J. W. (1950), Psychosurgery in the treatment of mental disorders and intractable pain. 2nd. Ed. Springfield, Ill.: Ch. C Thomas.
8. Handa, H., Mori, K., Yoshida, K., Stereoencephalotomy in agitated idiocy (cited by Sano).
9. Heimburger, R. F., Whitlock, C. C., Kalsbeck, J. E. (1966), Stereotaxic amygdalotomy for epilepsy with aggressive behaviour. J. Amer. med. Ass. *198*, 741—745.
10. Hess, W. R. (1947), Vegetative Funktionen und Zwischenhirn. Helv. Physiol. Acta Suppl. IV.
11. — (1969), Hypothalamus and thalamus: experimental documentation. Stuttgart: Thieme.
12. Ingram, W. R. (1952), Brain stem mechanisms in behaviour. EEG Clin. Neurophysiol. *4*, 397—406.
13. — Knott, J. R., Wheatly, M. D., Summer, T. D. (1951), Physiological relationships between hypothalamus and cerebral cortex. EEG Clin. Neurophysiol. *3*, 37—58.
14. Knight, G. (1964), The orbital cortex as an objective in the surgical treatment of mental illness. Brit. J. Surg. *51*, 114—124.
15. Kurotsu, T. (1954), Changes of finer structures of different gland cells indiced by the electrical stimulation of the hypothalamus. Med. J. Osaka Univ. *5*, 87—104.
16. Lebeau, J. (1954), Anterior cingulectomy in man. J. Neurosurg. *11*, 268—276.
17. Leksell, L. (1949), A stereotaxic apparatus for intracerebral surgery. Acta Chir. Scand. *99*, 229—233.
18. — (1971), Stereotaxis and radiosurgery. An operative system. Springfield, Ill.: Ch. C Thomas.
19. Narabayashi, H., Nagao, T., Saito, T., Yoshida, M., Naghata, M. (1963), Stereotaxic amygdalotomy for behaviour disorders. Arch. Neurol. (Chic.) *9*, 1—16.
20. Sano, K. (1954), Cingulectomy in the treatment of agitated mental defectives. Brain and Nerve *6*, 146—156.
21. — (1957), Fornicotomy Fol. psychiat. neurol. Jap. Suppl. *5*, 57—58.
22. — (1962), Sedative neurosurgery with special reference to posteromedial hypothalamotomy. Neurol. med. chir. *4*, 112—142.
23. — (1966), Sedative Stereoencephalotomy: Fornicotomy, upper mesencephalic reticulotomy and postero-medial hypothalamotomy. In: Progress in brain Research. 21 B Part B Clinical Studies. Ed.: Tokizane, T., Schade, J. P. Amsterdam: Elsevier.
24. — Mayanagi, Y., Sekino, H., Ogashiwa, M., Ishijima, B. (1970), Results of stimulation and destruction of the posterior hypothalamus in man. J. Neurosurg. *33*, 689—707.
25. Schvarcz, J. R., Driollet, R., Rios, E., Betti, O. (1972), Stereotactic hypothalamotomy for behaviour disorders. J. Neurol. Neurosurg. Psychiat. *35*, 356—359.
26. Scoville, W. B. (1949), Selective cortical undercutting as means of modifying and studying frontal lobe functions in man. Preliminary report of 43 operative cases. J. Neurosurg. *6*, 65—73.
27. Spiegel, E. A., Wycis, H. T., Freed, H. (1949), Thalamotomy: neuropsychiatric aspects. New York S. J. Med. *49*, 2273—2274.

28. Spiegel, E. A., Wycis, H. T., Freed, H., Orchinik, C. (1953), Thalamotomy and hypothalamotomy for the treatment of psychoses. Ass. Res. Nerv. Ment. Dis. *31*, 379—391.
29. Vaernet, K., Madsen, A. (1970), Stereotaxic amygdalotomy and basofrontal tractotomy in psychotics with aggressive behaviour. J. Neurol. Neurosurg. Psychiat. *33*, 858—863.

Author's address: Dr. V. E. Arjona, "Las Villas", Avda. M. Sinot s/n, Sevilla, Spain.

Section IV

Stereotactic Techniques

Acta Neurochirurgica, Suppl. 21, 195—209 (1974)
© by Springer-Verlag 1974

Department of Neurosurgery and Neuroradiology, Karolinska Sjukhuset,
Stockholm, Sweden

Stereotactic Radiosurgery in Intracranial Arterio-Venous Malformations

L. Steiner, L. Leksell, D. M. C. Forster, T. Greitz, and E.-O. Backlund

With 13 Figures

Abstract

Stereotactic radiosurgery has been used to treat five arteriovenous malformations, in which surgical excision could not be carried out, using the ^{60}Co Gamma Unit.

The malformation could no longer be seen at angiography performed in the first case at 19 and 36 months and in another case one year after therapy.

In the remainder 3 cases, no changes have been observed so far, but in two of them only one of several feeding arteries had been irradiated.

Introduction

At present direct intracranial surgery with excision is the treatment of choice for arterio-venous malformations, whenever possible. However, if factors exist contra-indicating craniotomy the neurosurgeon should be prepared to seek alternative methods of treatment. Conventional X-ray therapy has been tried in the past but generally abandonned. (Magnus 1921, Cushing and Bailey 1928, Ray 1941, Krayenbühl 1954, Potter 1955, Peterson and McKissock 1956, Olivecrona and Riives 1958, Svien and Peserico 1960, Pool 1965, French and Chou 1969, Johnson 1969.) More recently the possibilities of artificial embolization (Luessenhop and Spence 1960, Luessenhop 1969) or thrombosis (Taren and Gabrielsen 1970) as well as intimal hypertrophy provoked by cryosurgery (Walder et al. 1970, Walder 1971) have been explored and tested clinically.

The present report is part of a clinical and experimental study in progress on the effect of radiosurgery on intracranial vascular lesions.

In five cases of arterio-venous malformations a single dose of 5000 rads was administered to the aneurysm or to the feeding arteries using the

13*

Leksell stereotaxic system and narrow beams from the ⁶⁰Co Gamma Unit. (Leksell 1951, Leksell 1968, Leksell 1971).

The technique, some preliminary observations and problems arising from the use of radiosurgery for vessel pathology are presented.

Method and Material

After the initial diagnostic rapid serial angiography the procedure includes the following steps:

1. The coordinate frame is fixed to a cap of plaster of Paris or plastic applied to the patient's head.

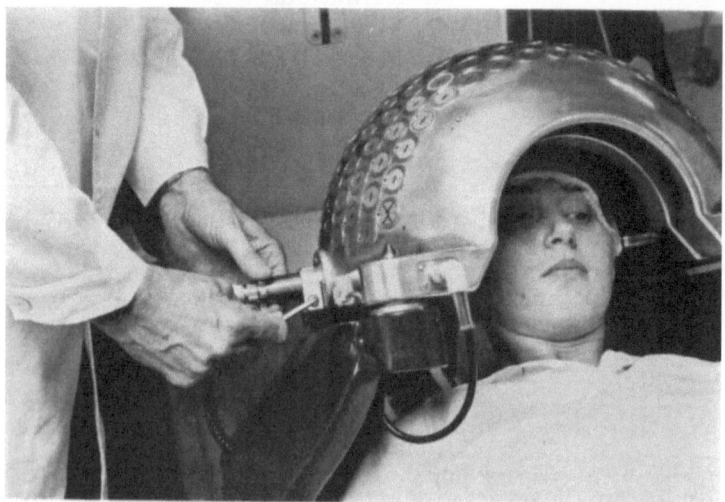

Fig. 1. The head of the patient is positioned according to the Z coordinate of the target

2. Stereotaxic angiography of the region harbouring the aneurysm is performed.

3. Two small bearings for the axis rods of the collimator helmet are embedded in the plaster corresponding to the X and Y coordinates of the target.

4. The lateral position of the head in the apparatus corresponds to the Z coordinate of the target (Fig. 1).

The beam cross-section is selected according to the size of the lesion required, and one single, or several combined, radiation fields are centered on the target. If the aneurysm is small it can be completely covered by one or more fields of radiation. If the malformation is larger the beams are directed on to the feeding arteries close to the lesion.

It is usually possible to include several pathological vessels in a single radiation field. Fig. 2 shows examples of the isodose configurations used. The procedure can be performed without general anesthesia.

Angiography, brain scanning, EEG and clinical controls were carried out in all patients at predetermined intervals after operation.

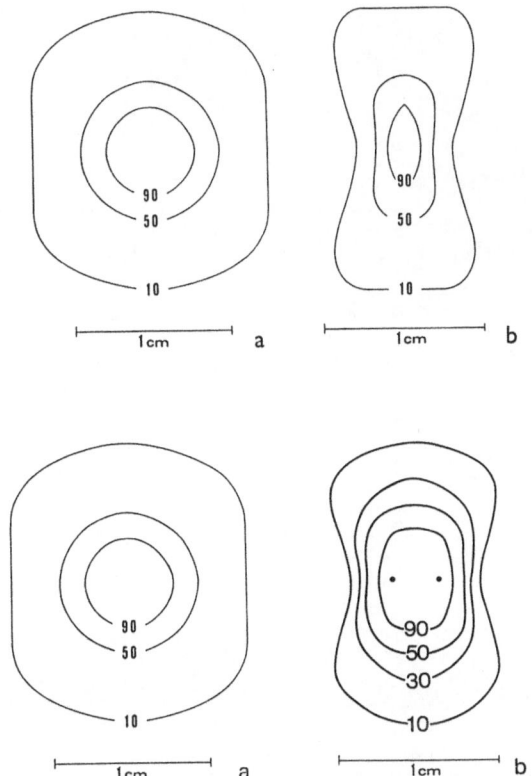

Fig. 2. Isodose configurations, simple and combined. Frontal (a) and lateral (b) views giving the percentage of the maximum radiation dose

Results

Case 1. E. A. B. The first patient was a 69-year old man with hypertension and chronic nephritis, admitted to our department in December 1969, after a subarachnoid haemorrhage. He had no neurological deficits apart from a transient superior homonymous quadrantic hemianopsia.

Angiography revealed a large arterio-venous malformation in the medial part of the left occipital lobe fed by the dilated posterior cerebral artery. The malformation and the feeding artery filled only from the vertebrobasilar system (Fig. 3).

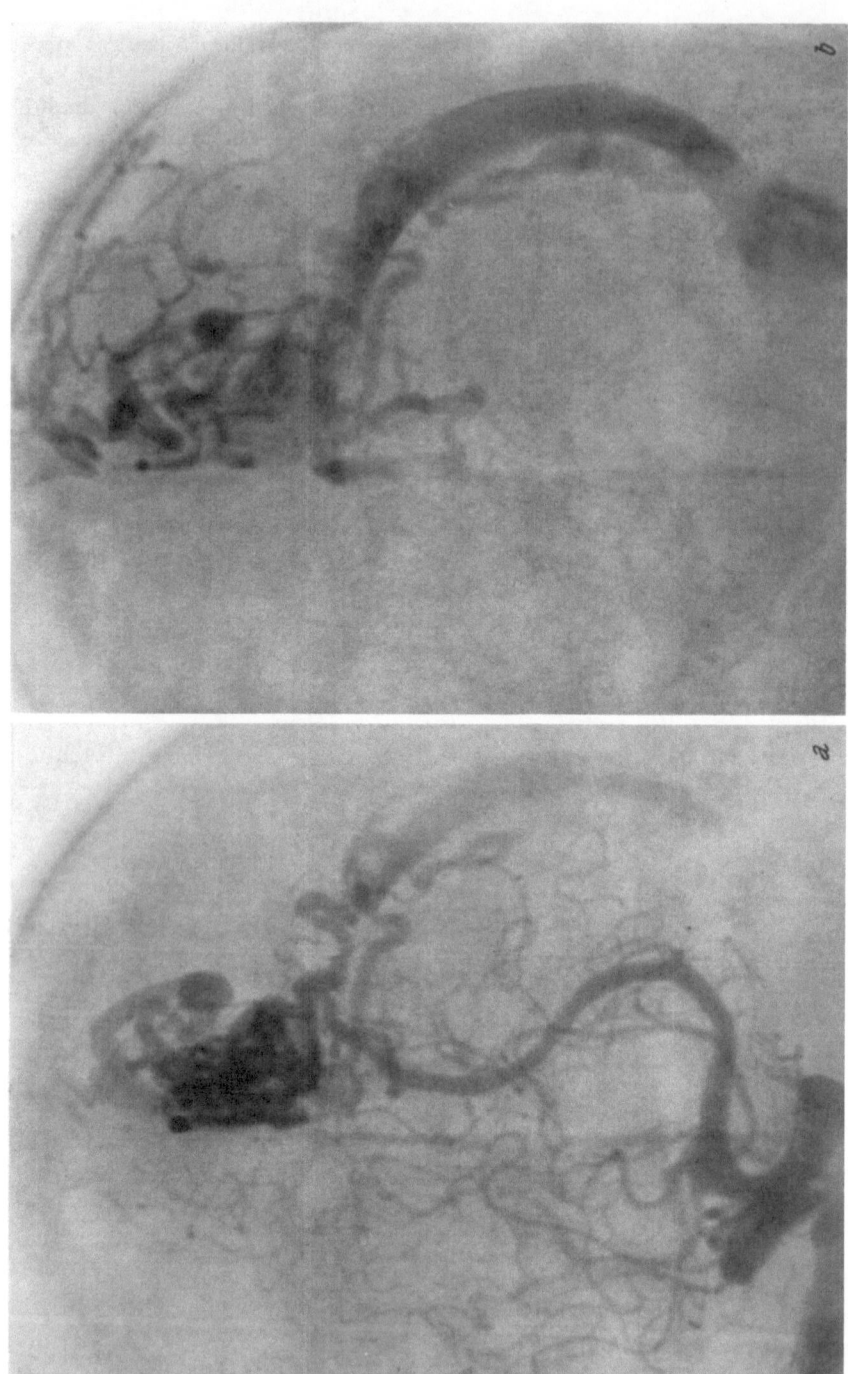

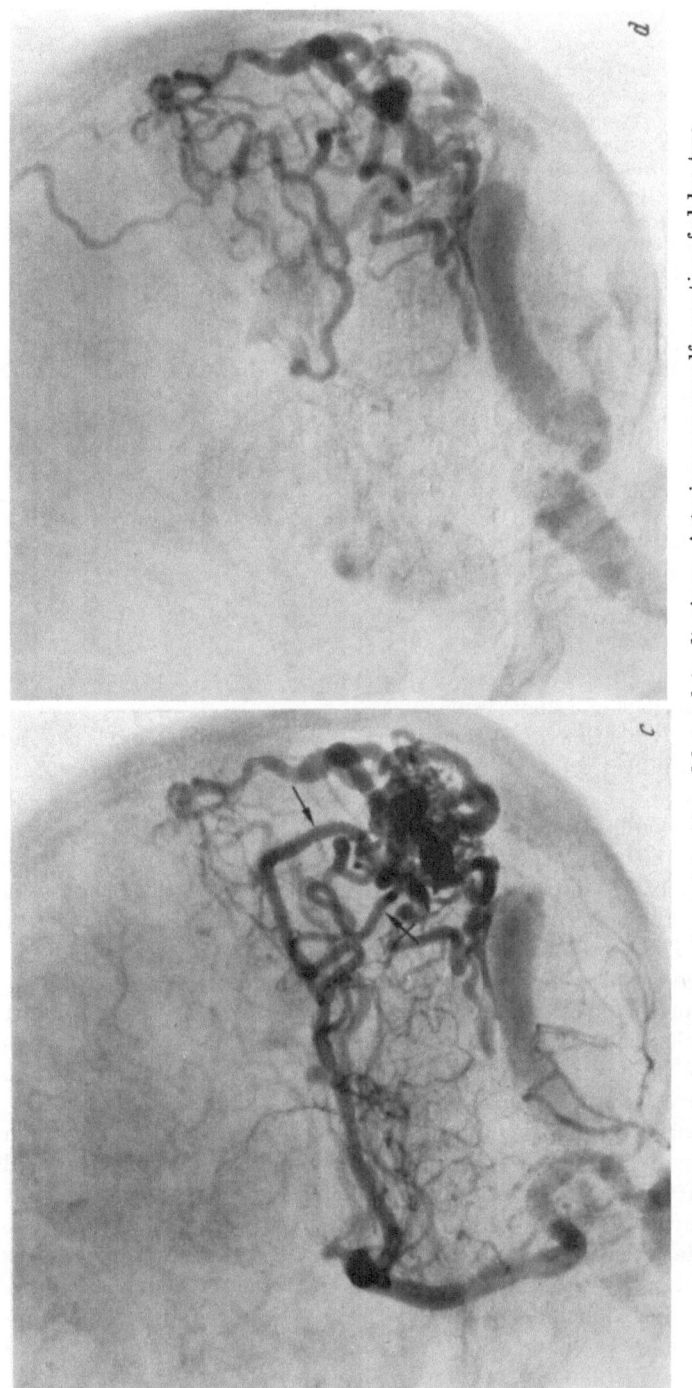

Fig. 3. Vertebral angiography, frontal (a, b) and lateral (c, d) views. Arteriovenous malformation fed by two branches (arrows) of the posterior cerebral artery. (Reproduced by courtesy of Acta Chir. Scand.)

Radiosurgery was performed in March 1970, and the target point located so that the two terminal branches of the feeding artery were included in the 50% isodose curve (Fig. 4). A single radiation field was used and 5000 rads given over a period of about half an hour.

The malformation remained unchanged until November 1971, when the angiograms no longer visualized the malformation and the feeding vessels were obliterated (Fig. 5). The obstructed segments coincided precisely with the preoperatively determined target point.

Case 2. S. E. A 10-year old girl was referred from another neurosurgical unit when angiography, following a subarachnoid haemorrhage, revealed a small arterio-venous malformation in the right basal ganglia (Figs. 6a, b).

At radiosurgery in April 1972 angiography showed that the lesion had increased slightly in size (Figs. 7a, b). A single dose of 5 krads was delivered so that the cluster of pathological vessels was almost completely covered. 4 months later angiography showed that the malformation had become markedly reduced in size (Figs. 8a, b).

Subsequent angiography, after 3 years in case 1 and after 1 year in case 2 showed no filling at all of either malformation, while in the remainder no changes have been observed so far.

Discussion

This appears to be the first occasion that stereotaxically directed Gamma rays have been used to obtain obliteration in arterio-venous malformations and aneurysms.

This application of radiosurgery although inspired by early radiotherapy, differs from it in principle and technique and above all in precision.

In the publications on radiotherapy in arterio-venous malformations published hitherto (Table 1) the details of treatment were often lacking, the fields of irradiation approximate and accuracy in dosimetry usually absent. Furthermore the doses were often low and given over a long period. The results were usually based on clinical criteria and follow-up with angiography, if done at all, was unsystematic.

The present method allows exact information on dose, volume, time and localization. It is hoped that the careful planning of the follow-up will give basic information on the interval between the radiation and the appearance of obliteration.

Our observations suggest the possibility that radiation may induce obliteration in vascular lesions and are in line with pathological studies in recent years concerning the early and late changes in the wall of vessels after radiation (Berdjis 1960, Smith 1961, Casarett 1968).

The fact that, the site of obliteration of the feeding vessels in case 1 coincided precisely with the predetermined target point makes a spontaneous obliteration independent of the radiosurgical procedure improbable. The early changes described in case 2 also coincided with the planned target, the malformation being the only one in this series small

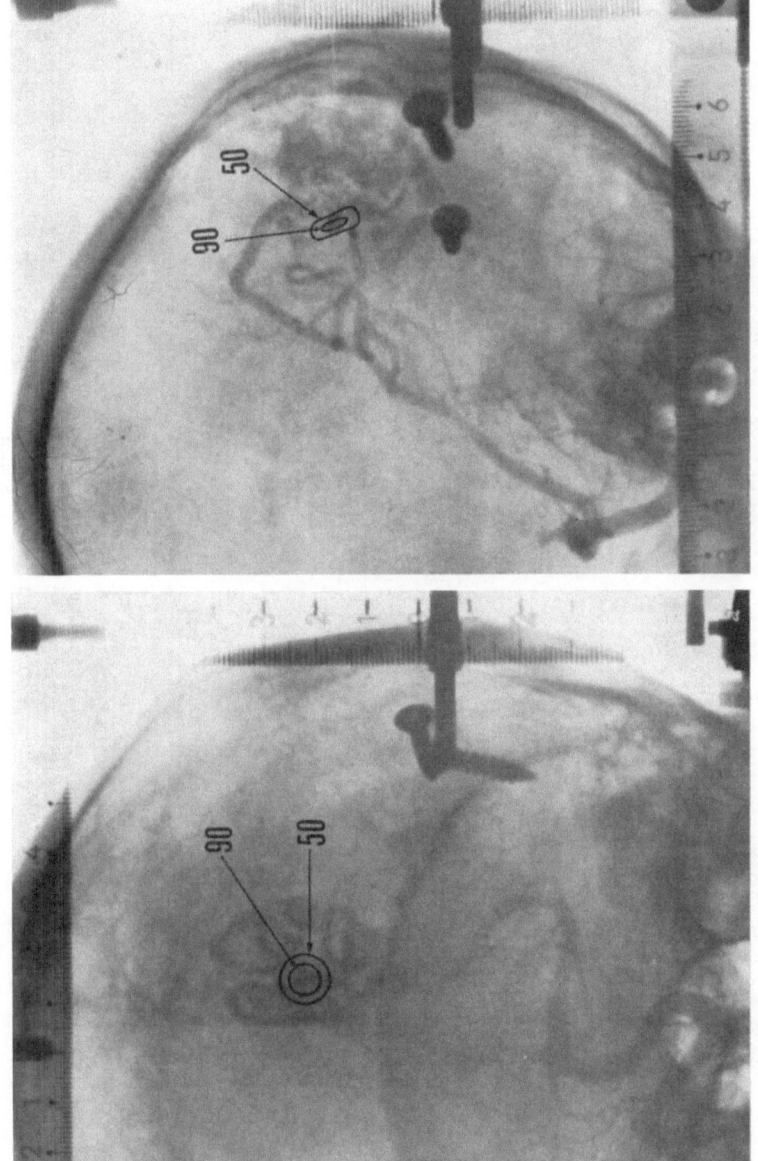

Fig. 4. Frontal (a) and lateral (b) views. Stereotaxic vertebral angiography on the day of radiosurgery. The 50% isodose curve includes the two feeding arteries. (Reproduced by courtesy of Acta Chir. Scand.)

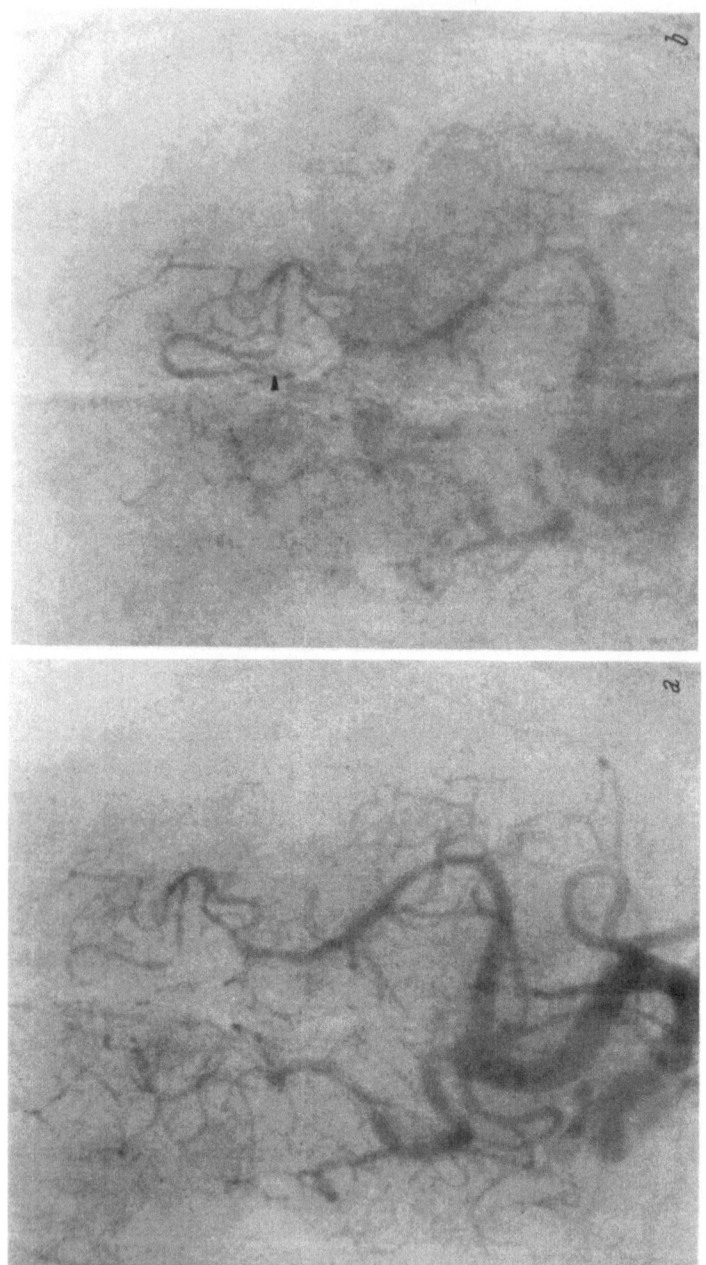

Fig. 5 a, b

Fig. 5. Vertebral angiogram 19 months after treatment showing no filling of the aneurysm. The posterior cerebral artery has returned to normal size and the two feeding arteries (arrows) show a slow circulation and a local constriction corresponding to their course through the target area. Contrast medium remains in these arteries during the capillary and venous phases. There is ordinary contrast filling of the intradural sinuses bilaterally. (Reproduced by courtesy of Acta Chir. Scand.)

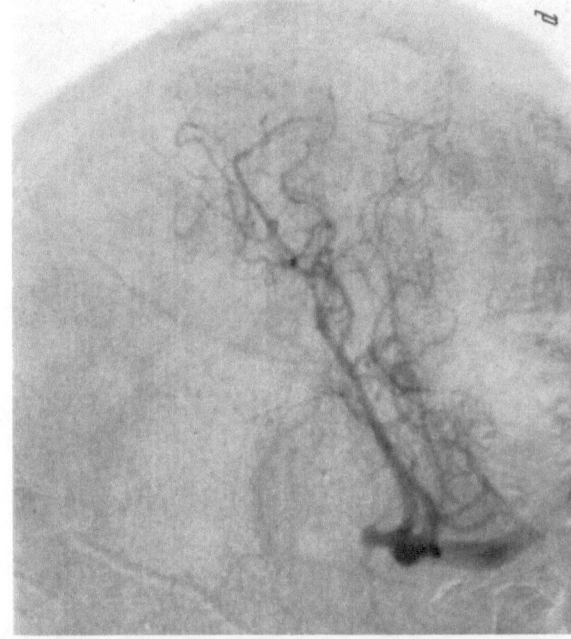

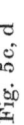

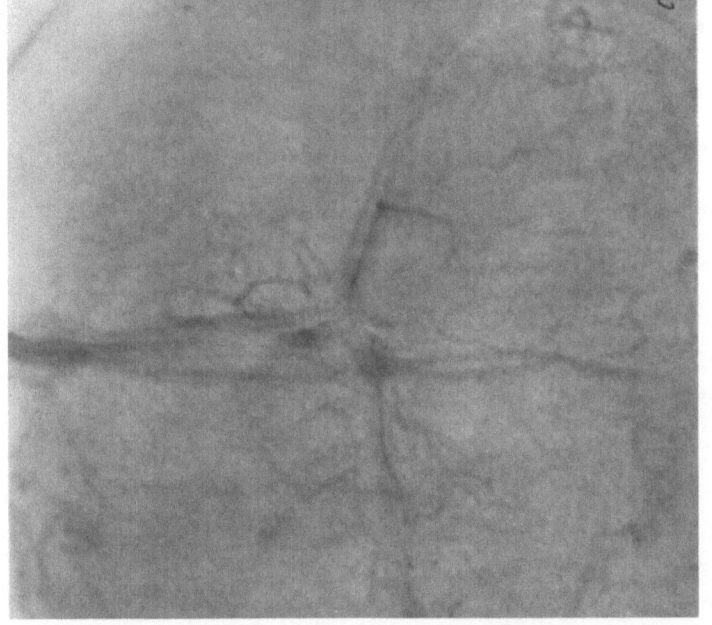

Fig. 5c, d

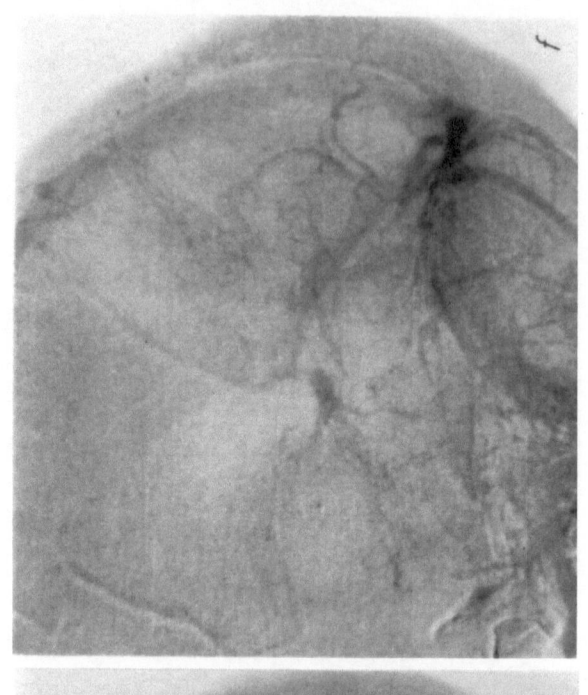

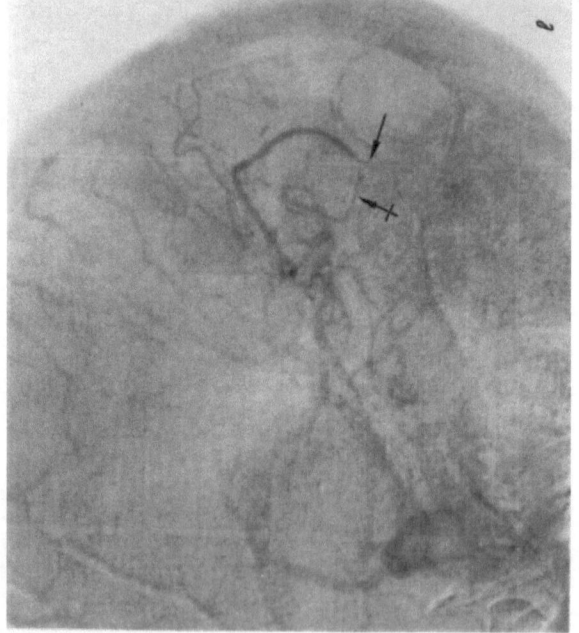

Fig. 5e, f

Table 1. *Publications on Conventional X-Ray Therapy in Arterio-Venous Malformations*

No.	Author	Year	Cases	Radiation type	Dose krad	Time	Volume	Follow-up Years	Follow-up Method
1	Magnus, U.	1921	1	radium	2	fraction repeated	?	7	clinical
2	Marque, A. M.	1927	2	X-ray	2	fraction repeated	?	?	clinical
3	Cushing, H. Bailey, P.	1928	8	X-ray	2	fraction repeated	?	>3	clinical operative
4	Ray, B. S.	1941	3	X-ray	3–13	fraction repeated	?	>3	clinical
5	Krayenbühl, H.	1954	4	X-ray	?	fraction repeated	?	3	angiography
6	Potter, J. M.	1955	10	X-ray radium	?	fraction repeated	?	up to 22	clinical
7	Peterson, J. H. McKissok, W.	1956	11	X-ray radium	?	fraction repeated	?	up to 14	clinical
8	Oliveerona, H. Riives, I.	1958	?	X-ray radium	?	fraction repeated	?	10	angiography clinical
9	Svien, H. J. Peserico, I.	1960	1	X-ray radium	3.7	fraction repeated	?	8	angiography
10	Pool, J. L.	1965	?	X-ray radium	?	fraction repeated	?	?	clinical angiography
11	Johnson, R. T.	1969	1	X-ray radium	?	fraction repeated	?	6	angiography
12	French, L. A. Chou, S. N.	1969	>6	X-ray radium	?	fraction repeated	?	2	clinical angiography

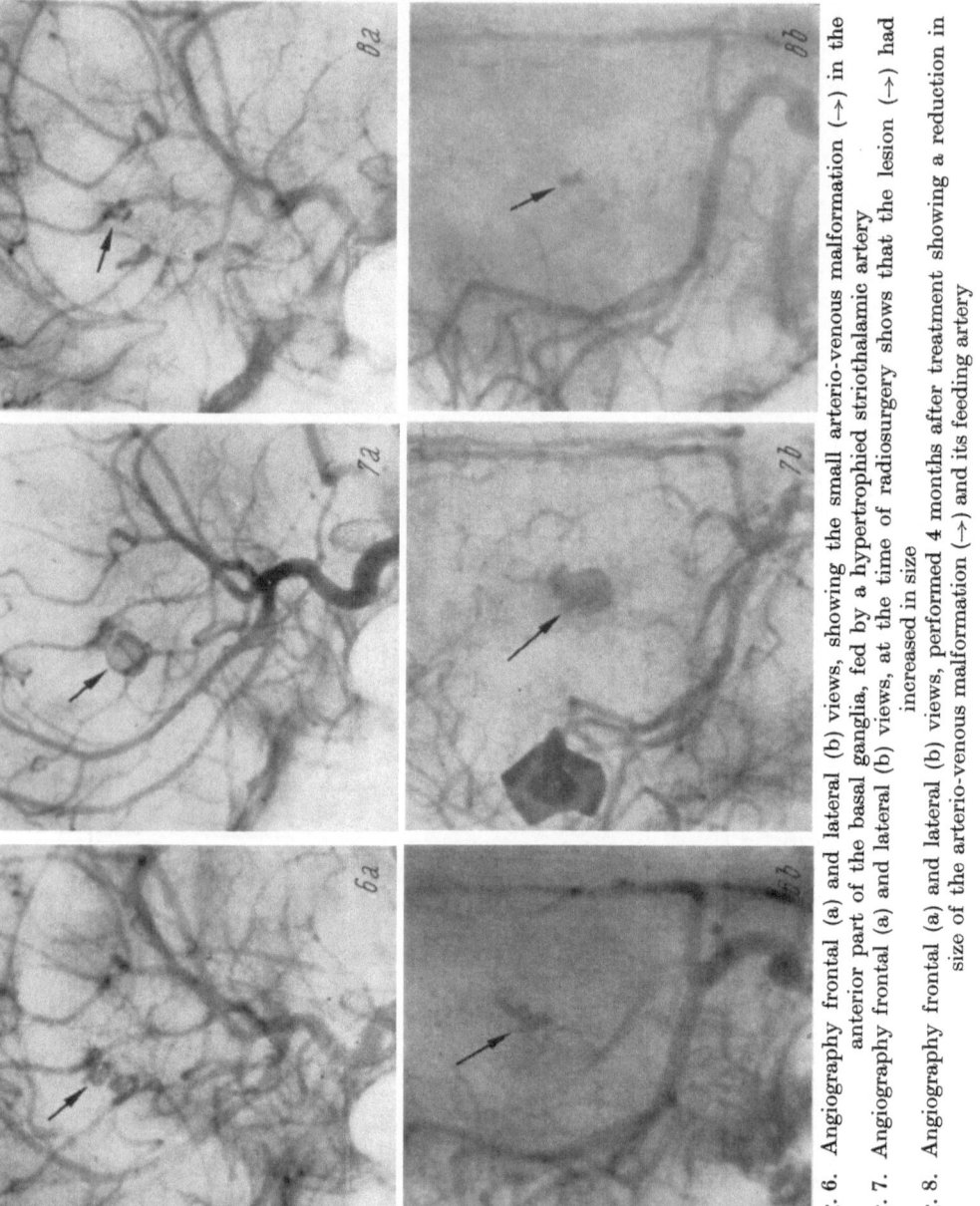

Fig. 6. Angiography frontal (a) and lateral (b) views, showing the small arterio-venous malformation (→) in the anterior part of the basal ganglia, fed by a hypertrophied striothalamic artery

Fig. 7. Angiography frontal (a) and lateral (b) views, at the time of radiosurgery shows that the lesion (→) had increased in size

Fig. 8. Angiography frontal (a) and lateral (b) views, performed 4 months after treatment showing a reduction in size of the arterio-venous malformation (→) and its feeding artery

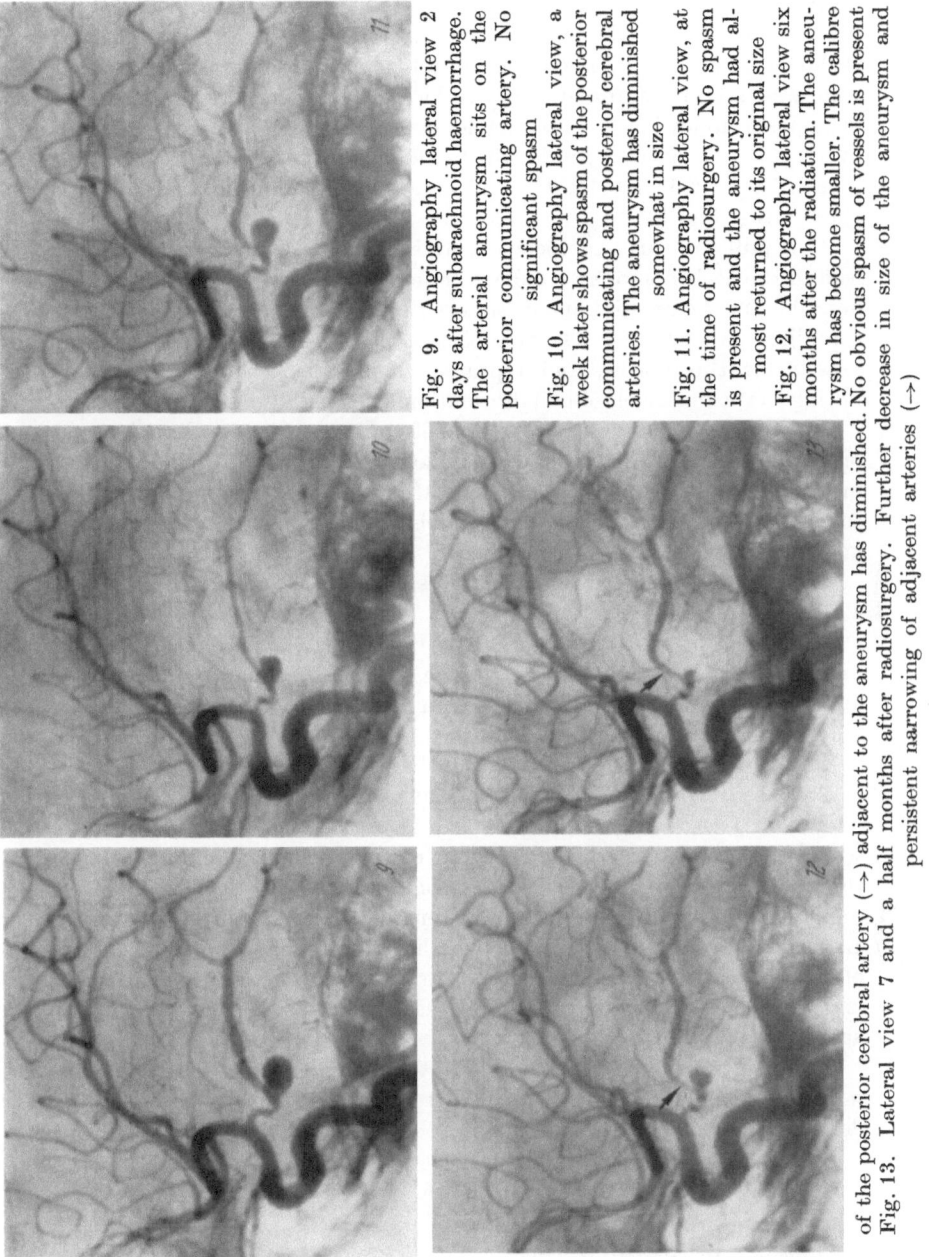

Fig. 9. Angiography lateral view 2 days after subarachnoid haemorrhage. The arterial aneurysm sits on the posterior communicating artery. No significant spasm

Fig. 10. Angiography lateral view, a week later shows spasm of the posterior communicating and posterior cerebral arteries. The aneurysm has diminished somewhat in size

Fig. 11. Angiography lateral view, at the time of radiosurgery. No spasm is present and the aneurysm had almost returned to its original size

Fig. 12. Angiography lateral view six months after the radiation. The aneurysm has become smaller. The calibre of the posterior cerebral artery (→) adjacent to the aneurysm has diminished. No obvious spasm of vessels is present

Fig. 13. Lateral view 7 and a half months after radiosurgery. Further decrease in size of the aneurysm and persistent narrowing of adjacent arteries (→)

enough to be virtually completely covered by the stereotactic lesion. Further evidence of the effect of radiation on pathological vasculature is shown by an arterial aneurysm (in a 61-year old hypertensive woman who was stuporose for several weeks from the ischaemic effects of vasospasm following a subarachnoid haemorrhage) treated by two overlapping fields of 5 krads which was much diminished in size after 6 months Figs. 9, 10, 11, 12, and almost completely obliterated after 7.5 months (Fig. 13).

It is still too early to speculate about the exact mechanisms which lead to the occlusion of an irradiated aneurysm. However, if the changes described in the arterial aneurysm are due to radiation, it would suggest a proliferative process. The role of age, the propensity of pathological vessels for thrombosis, and repeated small haemorrhages, in contributing to the occlusion of a malformation after radiation, are not known.

It is difficult to evaluate the risk of rupture in an irradiated vessel on the basis of our small material. However, no rupture has occurred in this series of patients, nor in 8 cats after receiving from 5 to 20 krads to the carotid artery nor in a rat which received 40 krads to the aorta and inferior vena cava.

In fact, hitherto, no complications have been observed in up to 42 months of follow-up.

The potential damage to the blood-brain barrier is perhaps of minor importance considering the small size of the lesion and the changes already present in the brain tissue surrounding the aneurysm.

Two major drawbacks remain:

1. The length of the latent period before the obliteration.

2. The risk of incomplete or excessive obliteration.

The first is of extreme importance in cases of arterial aneurysm in which the greatest risk for rebleeding exists in the first month after a subarachnoid haemorrhage. The second drawback is common to all methods aiming at obliteration by embolization or thrombotization. Experimental studies may show whether the latency and final extent of the obliterative process can be controlled by variations in dose, rate and volume as well as by the possible use of pharmacological or physical adjuvants.

The place of this method, if any, in the management of arteriovenous malformations and perhaps even arterial aneurysms remains to be determined.

References

1. Berdjis, C. C., et al. (1960), Cardiovascular system and radiation: -late effects of X-rays on the arteries of the adult. Strahlentherapie *112*, 595—602.
2. Cushing, H., Bailey, P. (1928), Tumours arising from the blood vessels of the brain. Springfield, Ill.: Ch. C Thomas.

3. French, L. A., Chou, S. N. (1969), Conventional methods of treating intracranial arterio-venous malformations. Progr. neurol. Surg. *3*, 274—319, Basel: Karger.
4. Johnson, R. T. (1969), Surgery of cerebral haemorrhage. In Recent advances in neurology and neuropsychiatry, pp. 102—128. London: Churchill.
5. Krayenbühl, H. (1954), Fifth int. Neurol. Congr. (Lisbon 1953) *3*, 173—178.
6. Leksell, L. (1951), The stereotaxic method. Acta Chir. Scand. *102*, 316—319.
7. — (1958), Cerebral radiosurgery. Acta Chir. Scand. *134*, 585—595.
8. — (1971), Stereotaxis and radiosurgery; an operative system, pp. 92. Springfield, Ill.: Ch. C Thomas.
9. Luessenhop, A. J., Spence, W. T. (1960), Artifical embolization of cerebral arteries. Report of use in a case of arteriovenous malformation. JAMA *172*, 1153—1155.
10. — (1969), Artificial embolization for cerebral arteriovenous malformations. Progr. Neurol. Surg. *3*, 320—362. Basel: Karger and Chicago: Year Book Publishers.
11. Magnus, V. (1921), Bidrag til hjernechirurgiens klinik og resultater, 138 pp. Kristiania: Merkur.
12. Olivecrona, H., Riives, I. (1958), Arteriovenous aneurysms of the brain. Arch. Neurol. (Chic.) (formerly AMA Arch. Neurol.) *59*, 567—602.
13. Peterson, J. H., McKissock, W. (1956), A clinical survey of intracranial angiomas with special reference to their mode of progression and surgical treatment: a report of 110 cases. Brain *79*, 233—266.
14. Pool, J. L. (1965), Aneurysms and arterio-venous anomalies of the brain. Diagnosis and treatment. New York: Hoeber Medical Division of Harper and Row.
15. Potter, J. M. (1955), Angiomatous malformations of the brains; their nature and prognosis. Ann. Roy. Coll. Surg. (Engl.) *16*, 227—243.
16. Ray, B. S. (1941), Cerebral arterio-venous aneurysms. Surg. Gynec. Obstet. *73*, 614—648.
17. Rubin, Ph., Casarett, W. (1968), Clinical radiation pathology, pp. 1057. Philadelphia: W. B. Saunders Comp.
18. Smith, D. J. (1961), Effects of gamma radiation on isolated surviving arteries and their vasa-vasorum. Amer. J. Physiol. *201*, 901—904.
19. Steiner, L., et al. (1972), Stereotaxic radiosurgery for cerebral arterio-venous malformations. Acta Chir. Scand. *138*, 459—464.
20. Svien, H. J., Peserico, I. (1960), Regression in size of arterio-venous anomaly. J. Neurosurg. *17*, 493—496.
21. Taren, J. A., Gabrielsen, T. O. (1970), Radio-frequency thrombosis of vascular malformations with a transvascular magnetic catheter. Science *168*, 138—141.
22. Walder, H. A. (1971), Application of cryotherapy in arterio-venous aneurysms. An experimental and clinical study. J. Neurol. Neurosurg. Psychiat. *34*, 105.
23. — Jaspar, H. H. J., Meijer, E. (1970), Application of cryotherapy in cerebrovascular anomalies. J. Psychiatr. Neurol. Neurochir. *73*, 471—486.

Authors' address: Dr. L. Steiner, Department of Neurosurgery and Neuroradiology, Karolinska Sjukhuset, Stockholm, Sweden.

Acta Neurochirurgica, Suppl. 21, 211—220 (1974)
© by Springer-Verlag 1974

Institute of Neurological Sciences and Department of Clinical Physics
and Bio-Engineering, Glasgow, Scotland

A Versatile Stereotaxic System Based on Cylindrical Co-Ordinates and Using Absolute Measurements

J. W. Turner and A. Shaw

With 9 Figures

Introduction

Stereotaxic instrumentation based on the rectangular co-ordinate system has been very fully developed, but the possible advantages of the cylindrical co-ordinate system (Turner 1972) appear to have been largely overlooked. We have developed such a system, which involves only modest modifications to the established instruments originally devised by Guiot (1958) and Gillingham (1960).

Requirements and Problems in Stereotaxic Instrumentation

Most would agree that the ideal characteristics of a stereotaxic system are that it should be accurate, easy to use, versatile in its application, comfortable for the patient and allow adequate observation and access to the patient. It should preferably not be unduly expensive. Absolute measurements are desirable as errors can arise from radiological magnification and distortion unless appropriate corrections are made in the methodology. The necessary corrections may involve expensive equipment or alterations to existing structures or systems (e.g. installation of teleradiology) or, alternatively, burdensome manoeuvres or calculations may become necessary. Since the target point itself is frequently not directly visible radiologically, it is commonly necessary to use intermediate radiological reference points. In these cases it is advantageous to have a simple way of relating the instrument to the target point via the intermediate radiological reference points in three dimensions. Rotational error due to malalignment between the co-ordinate system of the brain and that of the instrument, when using

14*

212   J. W. Turner and A. Shaw:

intermediate radiological reference points, may give rise to error (Mundinger 1967). The inevitable obligation to define a target point in three
dimensions is itself demanding, and particularly so when coupled with
the above various sources of error. Stereotaxic instruments seldom
fulfil all the above requirements or overcome the problems easily.

Cylindrical Co-Ordinate System

The present stereotaxic system is based on cylindrical co-ordinates
and uses absolute measurements. The cylindrical co-ordinate system
can be likened to a hat box on its side. The point of reference "O"

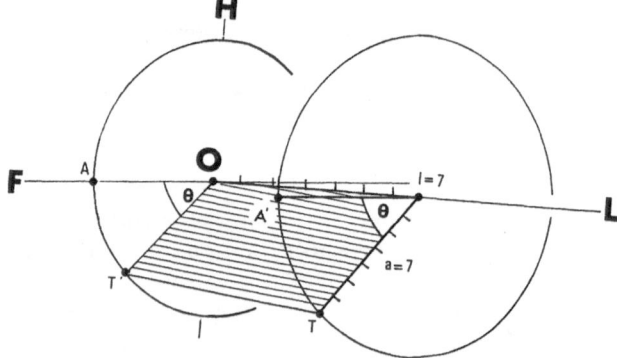

Fig. 1. Cylindrical co-ordinate system. *O* zero point of system, *T* target
point. Co-ordinates of T (l, a, $AOT' = \theta$)

of the system is located on the long axis of the cylinder which the hat
box represents, the target point is situated at a point on the rim of the
hat box. Thus, the target point "T" can be uniquely defined with respect
to "O" by two linear distances, namely, the depth "l" of the hat box
and the radius "a" of the hat box and by one angular measurement
"θ"—the angle made by the radius "a" with an initial reference line A'O.
In order to make use of the cylindrical co-ordinate system it is necessary
to be able to achieve angular measurements and to bring about precise
angular adjustments to the probe. This has been made possible by
incorporating a protractor into the type of instrument described by
Guiot (1958) and by Gillingham (1960). A linear scale has also been
included in order to measure radial distance. When coupled with a
two-dimensional mechanical analogue, a system has been developed which
achieves the requirements and overcomes the problems listed in the
previous section. The midline of the brain forms a natural and radiologically identifiable plane and can be made to correspond with one end

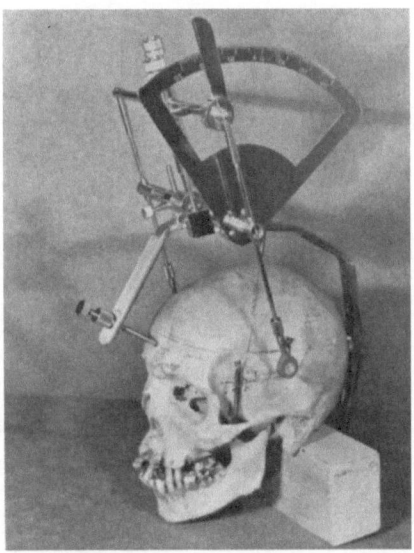

Fig. 2. Stereotaxic instrument of Gillingham with protractor modification

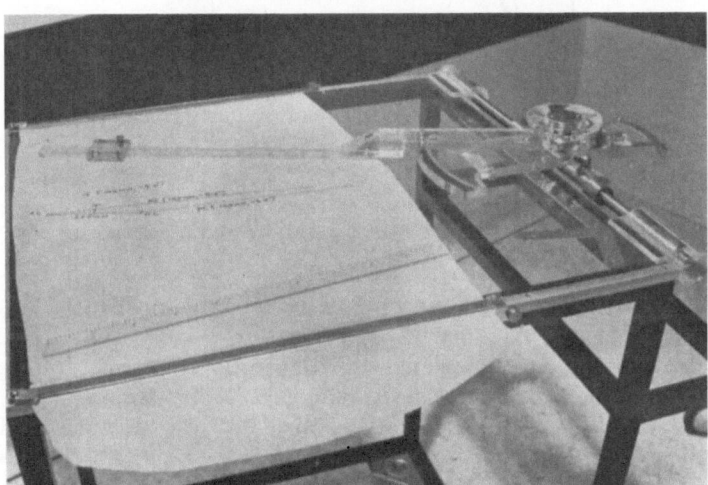

Fig. 3. Mechanical analogue

of the hat box of the cylindrical co-ordinate system. The sagittal bar
of the instrument is placed over this precise midline of the brain, as
described by Guiot and by Gillingham. Attached to the midline sagittal
bar of the instrument is a crossbar carrying a pair of radio-opaque
sights on two radial arms located on either side of the head. Each arm

represents the radius of the cylinder and can be rotated around its axis, and can also be extended or withdrawn so that the diameter of the cylinder can be varied. The distance "l" of the target point from the midline is obtained from a stereotaxic atlas in absolute terms and the probe can be set at this laterality on the stereotaxic instrument. This linear dimension having been dealt with, it is now possible to consider the system as a two-dimensional polar co-ordinate system in a para-

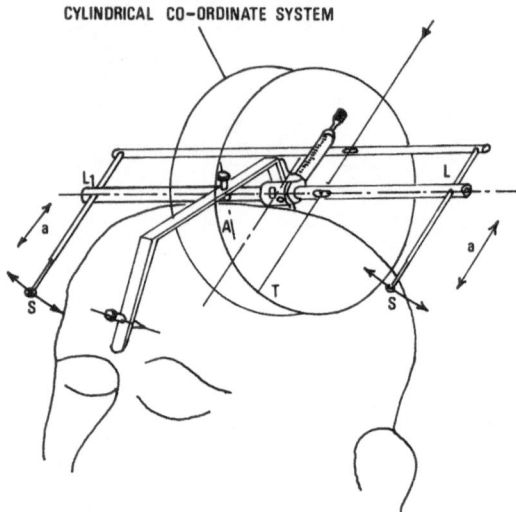

Fig. 4. Diagrammatic representation of the cylindrical co-ordinate system. *O* zero point of system, *T* target point, *SS* radio opaque sights

sagittal plane. The target can now be uniquely defined by the radius "a" and the angle "θ".

In practice, the sights are aligned with the aid of an image intensifier on the intermediate radiological reference point, for example, the anterior commissure. The radial distance "b" can now be read off directly from the instrument in absolute terms. From a lateral radiograph an angular measurement is obtained by the angle made between the line of the sight arms (o-Ac) and the reference line, i.e. the inter-commissural line (Ac-Pc). Since there is no magnification or distortion of angular measurement on the radiograph, provided the central beam of the X-rays is used, the angular measurement is also in absolute terms. From these two measurements, it is then possible to plot the inter-mediate radiological reference point on the two-dimensional mechanical analogue. Alternatively, the polar co-ordinates of both intermediate radiological reference points can be obtained from the instrument and then plotted on the analogue without the necessity of making the radiographic angular measurement. The absolute distance between the reference points can be directly measured on the analogue. The relationships of the target point and the intermediate radiological reference points are determined from the stereotaxic atlas and then plotted on the mechanical analogue. The polar co-ordinates of the target point are

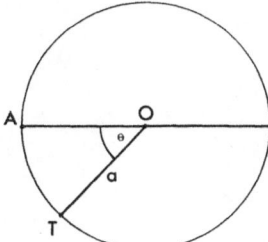

Fig. 5. Polar co-ordinates. O zero point of system, T target point. Co-ordinates of T (a, θ)

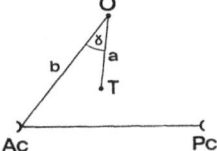

Fig. 6. Cylindrical co-ordinate system. The intermediate radiological reference points are plotted on the analogue from data obtained from the instrument. The target point is plotted from data obtained from the atlas. The co-ordinates of the target point are read from the analogue. O zero point of system, T target point, Ac intermediate radiological reference point

obtained by moving the sight arm analogue from the reference point to correspond with the plotted target point. The new radius "a" and the change in angle (i.e. "γ") can be read off the analogue and transferred to the instrument. The sights will, therefore, become automatically aligned on the target point and the probe can then be passed in the desired parasagittal plane (distance "l") along the radius "a" to the target point. Instead of the mechanical analogue, calculations using the cosine and sine laws can be used, or, alternatively again, a nomogram or computer programme can be used. However, the mechanical analogue is simple in construction and use and other methods seem hardly worth while. If it is necessary to reach a target very close to the midline, an oblique track can be used as previously described by Gillingham, without any alteration to the above system. With regard to the mechanical accuracy of the system, it can be shown that the predicted target point can be transferred from the mechanical analogue to the instrument

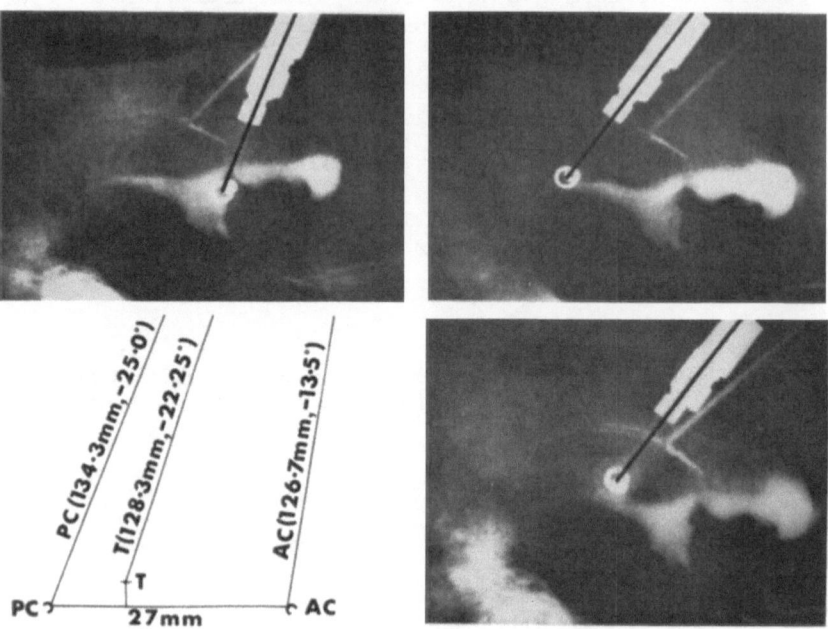

Fig. 7. Thalamotomy. Top left: sights aligned on anterior commissure, top right: sights aligned on posterior commissure, bottom left: anterior and posterior commissures plotted on analogue and co-ordinates of target thereby obtained, bottom right: sights aligned on the target point

with a reasonable degree of precision, in the order of 0.1 mm. A four times magnification was chosen for the analogue to correspond with that of the atlas of Schaltenbrand and Bailey.

Requirements of the System

It is imperative to define the midline and this is usually undertaken at the first of two stages in the surgical procedure (Gillingham). The midline is determined by outlining the fourth and third ventricles and also the septum pellucidum of the lateral ventricles with Conray (Methylglucamine iothalamate) or Myodil (Iophendylate) and air. It is imperative to define a reference line such as the intercommissural line. It is necessary to have an image intensifier available.

Applications

This system can be applied to a wide variety of targets within the central nervous system.

1. Thalamotomy: Thalamotomy in the treatment of Parkinsonism may be undertaken with the patient in a sitting position, under local anaes-

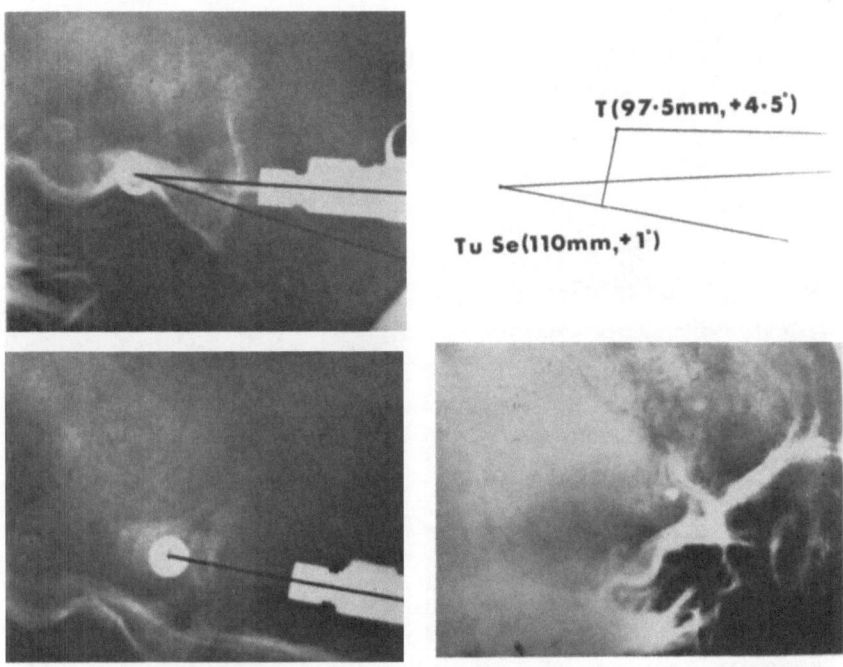

Fig. 8. Fronto-thalamic tractotomy. Top left: sights aligned on the tuberculum sellae (TuSe), top right: tuberculum sellae and target point plotted on analogue, bottom left: sights aligned on target point, bottom right: postoperative film showing four marker balls in line

thesia. After the sagittal bar of the instrument has been secured to the skull corresponding with the midline of the brain, Conray ventriculography is undertaken to define the anterior and posterior commissures, as the intermediate radiological reference points. With the help of the image intensifier, the sights of the instrument are aligned on the anterior commissure. The distance from the sights to the "O" zero point of the instrument (i.e. radius of the cylinder "b") can be read directly from the instrument. From a lateral radiograph the angle made between the sight arms and the intercommissural line is measured. These two measurements are then plotted on the mechanical analogue. Alternatively, the polar co-ordinates of the two commissures can both be plotted on the analogue. The relationship of the target point to the intermediate radiological reference points is established from the atlas and plotted on the analogue. The sight arm analogue is then moved to correspond with the target point itself, and the angle through which

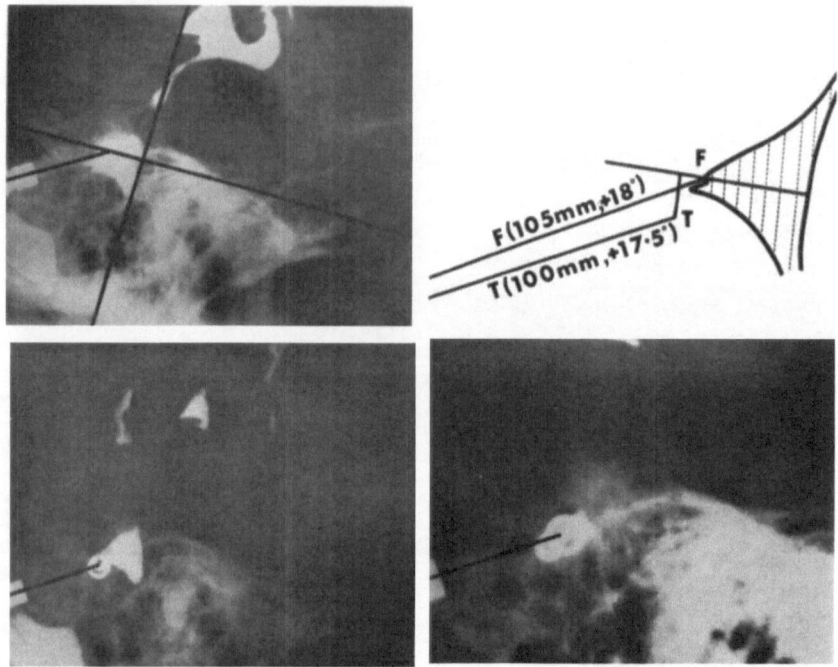

Fig. 9. Dentatotomy. Top left: sights aligned on fastigium, top right: fastigium F and target point plotted on analogue, bottom left: sights aligned on target point, bottom right: sights and marker ball after lesion making

the sight arms are moved and the distance through which they have to be retracted or extended can then be read off directly from the analogue and these polar co-ordinates transferred to the stereotaxic instrument. The probe can then be passed in the appropriate parasagittal plane to the target point. Physiological corroboration of the position of the probe is, of course, sought.

2. Stereotaxic Fronto-Thalamic Tractotomy: With the patient in the sitting or any other convenient position and under general anaesthesia, the sagittal bar is secured to the skull over the midline of the brain. The aim is to create a thin flat lesion as described by Knight (1965).

With the help of the image intensifier the target sights of the crossbar are then aligned on the tuberculum sellae. The orbital plate is used as the reference line. The radius of the cylinder is read off directly from the instrument. The angular measurement is taken from a lateral radiograph. The information is transferred to the mechanical analogue on which the relationship of the target point with the tuberculum sellae is established. The polar co-ordinates of the target point are then obtained from the analogue and transferred to the stereotaxic instrument.

3. Dentatotomy (Heimburger, Nashold, Siegfried, Zervas): With the patient in the supine position under general anaesthesia, the sagittal bar of the instrument is secured to the skull in the exact midline of the brain. With the help of the image intensifier and positive contrast ventriculography, the target sights are aligned on the fastigium of the fourth ventricle. The floor of the fourth ventricle is also defined. The radial distance "b" is obtained, the angular measurement between the sight arms aligned on the fastigium of the fourth ventricle, and a perpendicular dropped from it to the floor of the fourth ventricle can be measured on a lateral radiograph. The measurements are transferred to the analogue where the relationship of the dentate nucleus to the fastigium has already been established. The appropriate corrections in the radial distance and the angle are then transferred to the instrument.

Summary

We have described a stereotaxic system using cylindrical co-ordinates. This has been achieved (1) by incorporating a protractor into the type of instrument described by Guiot and by Gillingham, so that angular measurements can be made, and (2) by the help of a two-dimensional mechanical analogue. As with the instruments of Guiot and of Gillingham, no rotational error occurs and no extra expensive apparatus is required, provided that an image intensifier is available. It is reasonably comfortable for the patient, who is accessible to the surgeon. The system described is simple and accurate in practice. No calculations are required. Absolute measurements are used. The system is versatile in its application in stereotaxis and also in the path that may be selected for the probe track in approaching a target point.

References

1. Gillingham, F. J., Watson, W. S., Donaldson, A. A., Naughton, J. A. (1960), The surgical treatment of Parkinsonism. Brit. Med. J. *2*, 1395—1402.
2. Guiot, G. (1958), Le traitement des syndromes parkinsoniens par la destruction du pallidum interne. Neurochir. *1*, 94—98.

3. Heimburger, R. F. (1967), Dentatectomy in the treatment of dyskinetic disorders. Confin. Neurol. *29*, 101—106.
4. Knight, G. C. (1965), Stereotactic tractotomy in the surgical treatment of mental illness. J. Neurol. Neurosurg. Psychiat. *28*, 304—310.
5. Mundinger, F., Uhl, H. (1967), Investigations into possible roentgenographic errors in stereotaxis. Confin. Neurol. *29*, 202—207.
6. Nashold, B. S., Slaughter, D. G. (1969), Effects of stimulating or destroying the deep cerebellar regions in man. J. Neurosurg. *31*, 172—186.
7. Schaltenbrand, G., Bailey, P. (Eds.) (1959), Introduction to stereotaxis with an atlas of the human brain. Vol. I–III. Stuttgart: G. Thieme.
8. Siegfried, J. (1971), Stereotaxic cerebellar surgery. Int. Symp. Stereoencephalotomy, Bratislava.
9. Turner, J. W. (1972), Principles of stereotaxic instrumentation. Engineering in Medicine *1*, 98—103.
10. Zervas, N. T., Horner, F. A., Pickern, K. S. (1967), The treatment of dyskinesia by stereotaxic dentatectomy. Confin. Neurol. *29*, 93—100.

Authors' address: J. W. Turner, Institute of Neurological Sciences, Southern General Hospital, and A. Shaw, Department of Clinical Physics and Bio-Engineering, Glasgow, Scotland.

Acta Neurochirurgica, Suppl. 21, 221—226 (1974)
© by Springer-Verlag 1974

Neurosurgical Clinic (Prof. J. Bonnal) and Neuroanatomy Laboratory
(Prof. M. A. Gerebtzoff), University of Liège, Belgium

Serial Stereotaxic Biopsies

A. Waltregny, V. Petrov, and J. Brotchi

With 2 Figures

The accuracy of approach to various brain structures by the stereo-taxic method has induced some authors to do biopsy samplings (Housepian and Pool 1960–1962, Jinnai et al. 1961, Heath et al. 1961, Kalyanaraman and Gillingham 1964). Most of the techniques involve samplings by suction through a trocar (Housepian and Pool 1960–1962, Kalyanaraman and Gillingham 1964). A Silverman needle is more rarely used (Heath et al. 1961).

All the authors stress the good quality of the samples which can be studied by a conventional histological technique, a histochemical technique and even, if required, by electron microscopy. It is worthwhile noting, however, that the biopsies are considered as positive if they show nerve cells, and as negative if they only show some white substance (Housepian and Pool 1960). Finally, it must be noted, that some authors (Kalyanaram and Gillingham 1964), material may afford no interpretation in 10% of the samples, due to an excess of blood clots.

The increasing interest of interstitial stereotaxic radiotherapy of brain tumours, which are more or less inoperable by the conventional neurosurgical techniques (Mundinger 1966, Bancaud et al. 1970, Andrea 1971, Lindstrom 1971, Bonnal et Waltregny 1972), implies that the topographic limits of the tumour be accurately assessed and that a histological diagnosis be formally made.

Thus, after the radioisotopic, neuroradiological and electrophysiological localizations, the biopsies effected at various levels seem to be essential in order to define the actual extension and the exact nature of the tumour.

Material and Method

The stereotaxic technique used is that of Talairach and the particular modalities of its application in our unit have been reported elsewhere (Waltregny 1971).

Following the neuroradiological, stereotaxic and electrophysiological localizations of the tumour, and the superposition of cranial scintigraphs (also at a 1/1 scale), the coordinates of the trajectory of biopsy probes are calculated so as to approach the tumour by its largest presumed axes. By using the guiding systems of the frame, a 2.4 mm trephine hole is drilled and the Metzel-Wittmoser ventriculoscope forceps are inserted. The samplings are made centimetre by centimetre, and each sampling site is visualized by full-face and profile X-rays.

For basic histology, the biopsy fragments are fixed with 10% formol neutralized with chalk, for three days. Then they are coated with paraffin, and are cut into slices 5 microns thick. Two basic stains are always used: toluidine blue and hemalun-eosin. The study can then be completed using the other conventional histological techniques according to the problems encountered.

For the histochemical study, the fragments are put into carbon dioxide snow and are sliced, with the cryostat, to a thickness of 8–10 microns. The incubation is then made in an adequate substratum according to the dehydrogenase studied, and to which is added tetranitroblue of tetrazolium. One is thus able to study the dehydrogenases of glutamate, of glucose-6-phosphate, of isocitrate with a NAD or NADP coenzyme, of lactate and of its slow and rapid isoenzymes (Ant. a total of 7 enzymes). A portion of the biopsy fragment is fixed with brominized formol and sliced while frozen to a thickness of 20–25 microns, so as to stain the astrocytes according to Cajal's method.

Results and Discussion

Forty-two samples have thus been obtained from five patients, and the biopsies have been classified according to one, two or three trajectories. All fragments were of excellent quality and afforded a detailed histological diagnosis of the tumour and the correct assessment of its extension limits (Fig. 1 and Fig. 2). Moreover, this technique is now used for the histochemical study of epileptic foci which have been localized by stereoelectroencephalography (Figs. 1 e and f).

No puncture accident was observed, but it should be borne in mind that the trajectories of the sampling forseps are always calculated so as to avoid the vessels already localized by stereotaxic angiography. Moreover, as a safety measure, a heparinized trocar is always inserted to check the absence of bleeding after sampling (should bleeding actually occur,

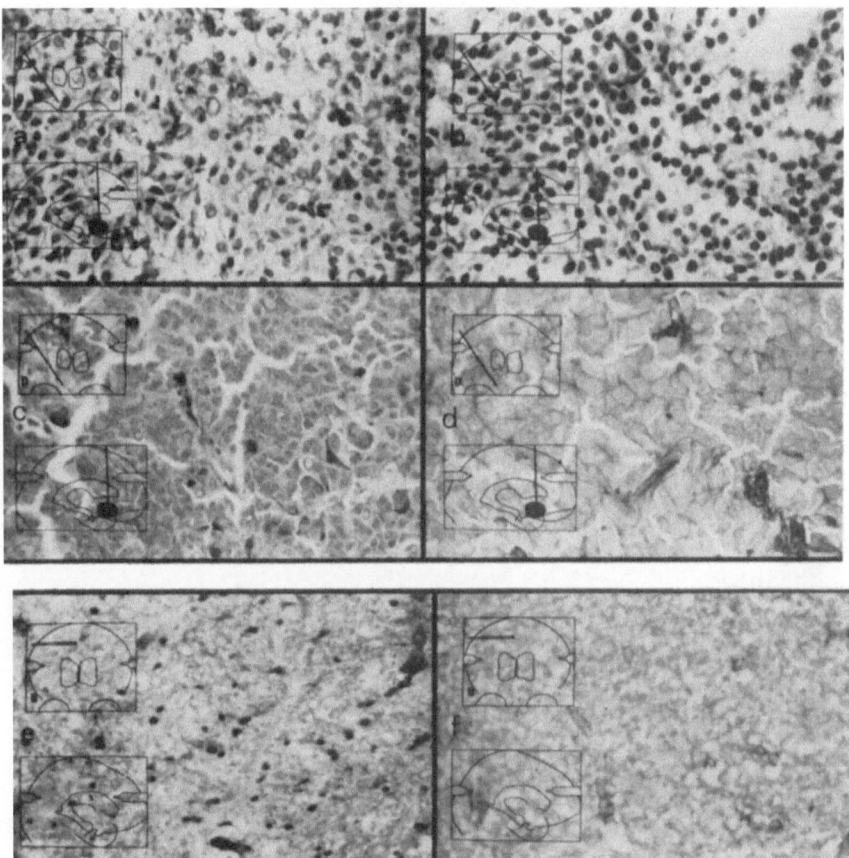

Fig. 1. a to d: sub-frontal tumour. Histological study of a sample (× 280). On the diagram, the grey-tinted area represents the sampling site with respect to the volume of the tumour as estimated by the neuroradiological study. a toluidine blue; numerous small tumoural cells, evocative of an ependymoma or of an adenoma, b hemalan-eosin of the same sample, c azan; chromophobe material with rare acidophilic cells, d PAS; hypophysial adenoma. Thus, contrary to the first hypothesis, the complementary stainings showed the existence of a chromophobe hypophysial adenoma. Surgery confirmed this diagnosis (a giant adenoma with no impairment of the field of vision). e and f: epileptic focus on the margin of a cortical exeresis; histochemical study (× 280). e Cajal's method; evidence of a few astrocytes and of numerous histiocytes, f iso S lactic dehydrogenase; no reactional astrocytes

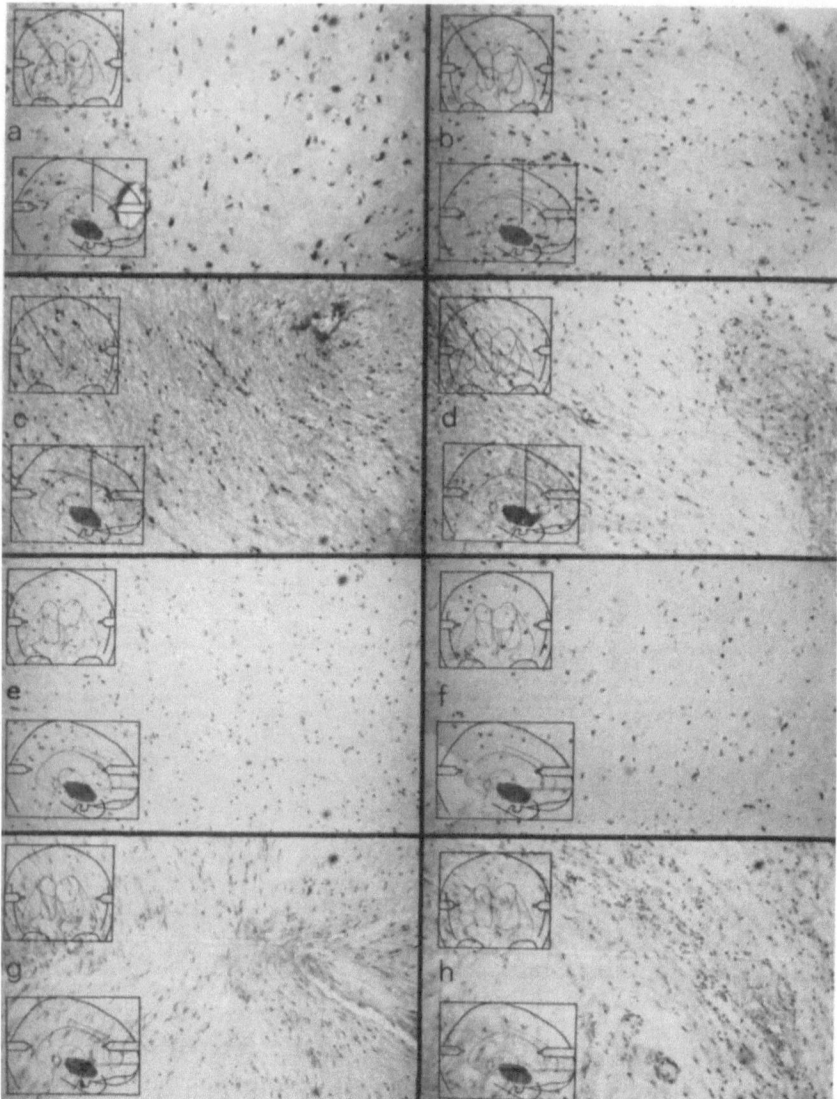

Fig. 2. Stereotaxic biopsies obtained at various levels according to two trajectories (×60). Right paraventricular tumour; histological diagnosis: spongioblastoma. (a to d) oblique trajectory: toluidine blue, (e to h) frontal trajectory: hemalan-eosin. On the diagram, the grey-tinted areas represent the sampling sites with respect to the volume of the tumour as estimated by the neuroradiological study. a white substance and some neurons of the caudate nucleus, b edge of the tumour, c tumour, d tumour, e white substance, f white substance, g tumour, h tumour. It can be seen that the anatomical and the radiological concordance is not perfect; in b the tumour is already histologically present; in f the tumour is not yet approached

coagulation at various levels could easily be carried out). No neurological after-effect has been reported.

The Metzel and Wittmoser forceps yielded better results than the Silverman needle we formerly used. The samples are of a larger volume, which is of considerable help for the histological study, especially when several staining techniques have to be used.

Summary

The authors present the results of cerebral biopsies, made centimetre by centimetre at various levels under stereotaxic conditions, in order to correctly assess the nature and volume of a tumour.

A conventional histological study and/or a histochemical study were carried out on the fragments thus obtained.

References

1. Andrea, d' F., de Divitiis, E., Signorelli, C. D., Cerillo, A. (1971), Stereotaxic implantation of radioisotopes in brain tumors. International Symposium of Stereoencephalotomy. Bratislava, 4–6 Juillet.

2. Bancaud, J., Talairach, J., Bordas-Ferrer, M., Bonis, A., Morel, P., Bresson, M., Amant, G. (1970), Intérêt de l'exploration SEEG des processus occupant de l'espace dans l'interprétation de l'EEG (rapport). XVII° Réunion Européenne d'enseignement électroencéphalographique. Marseille, 1–5 Septembre.

3. Bonnal, J., Waltregny, A. (1972), Diagnostic précoce et possibilités thérapeutiques des tumeurs cérébrales. Rev. Med. Liège 27, 120—122.

4. Heath, R. G., John, S., Foss, O. (1961), Stereotaxic biopsy. A method for the study of discrète brain regions of animals and man. Arch. Neurol. 4, 291—300.

5. Housepian, E. M., Pool, J. L. (1960), The accuracy of human stereoencephalotomy as judged by histological confirmation of roentgenographic localization. J. New Ment. Dis. 130, 520—525.

6. — — (1962), Application of stereotaxic methods to histochemical, electronmicroscopic and electrophysiological studies of human subcortical structures. Confin. Neurol. 22, 171—177.

7. Jinnai, D., Nisimoto, A., Matsumoto, K., Handa, S. (1961), Pallidotomy and thalamo-capsulotomy for parkinsonism. II int. Congr. Neurol. Surg. Washington D. C. 1961. Excerpta Med. 36, E 94, E 95.

8. Kalyanaraman, S., Gillingham, F. J. (1964), Stereotaxic biopsy. J. Neurosurg. 21, 854—858.

9. Lindstrom, P. A. (1971), A simplified stereotactic method for irradiation of larger subcortical structures. International Symposium of Stereoencephalotomy, Bratsilava, 4–6 Juillet.

10. Mundinger, F. (1966), The treatment of brain tumors with radioisotopes. Progr. neurol. Surg. Vol. 1, 202- -257. Basel-New York: Karger.

11. Talairach, J., Ruggiero, G., Aboulker, J., David, M. (1955), A new method of treatment of inoperable brain tumours by stereotaxic implantation of radioactive gold. A preliminary report. Brit. J. Radiol. 28, 62—74.
12. — Szikla, G., Bonis, A., Bancaud, J. (1963), Utilisation thérapeutique des isotopes radio-actifs en neurochirurgie. La Revue de Médecine 8, 1—9.
13. — — et al. (1967), Atlas stéréotaxique du télencéphale, 323 pp. Paris: Masson.
14. Waltregny, A. (1971), Neurochirurgie stéréotaxique et aire motrice supplémentaire. Prix de Neurochirurgie "Docteurs Paul et Philippe Martin". 113 pp. Bruxelles.

Authors' address: Dr. A. Waltregny, Clinique Neurochirurgicale, Hopital de Bavière, B-4000 Liège, Belgium.

Acta Neurochirurgica, Suppl. 21, 227—233 (1974)
© by Springer-Verlag 1974

Newcastle General Hospital, Newcastle upon Tyne, England,
The Midland Centre for Neurosurgery and Neurology, Smethwick, Warley,
Worcestershire, England

A Simple Method for Obtaining Stereotaxic Biopsies from the Human Basal Ganglia.
A Case of Cerebral Porphyria

J. Hankinson, P. Hudgson, G. W. Pearce, and C. J. Morris

With 6 Figures

The importance of the stereotactic method for obtaining small samples from pre-determined structures in the brain has been emphasized on numerous occasions although only a few studies have ensued. A simple method was described by Kalyanaraman and Gillingham in 1964 and in Newcastle upon Tyne more recently we developed a particularly simple instrument and technique which will remove a cylinder of tissue in a condition suitable for electron microscopy and in sufficient amount for most relevant biochemical analyses. The biopsy cannula is illustrated in Fig. 1 and consists of a tube 19.5 cms long with an outer diameter of 2 mm and an inner diameter of 0.7 mm. A stilette lies within the cannula extending to the sharpened tip. The instrument is introduced to a point 3–4 mm above the area to be examined when the stilette is removed from the cannula which is then introduced in a rotatory way with the isolation of a small cylinder of brain tissue. A three-way tap and syringe is then attached and a vacuum produced inside the cannula which holds the biopsy in place while the instrument is withdrawn from the patient and stereotaxic frame. The biopsies are expressed gently into fixative for electron microscopy by slight air pressure from the syringe; alternatively, they can be frozen for biochemical studies or otherwise prepared.

The instrument was tested in the monkey brain to determine what structural artifacts are produced by the procedure at the electron micro-

J. Hankinson et al.:

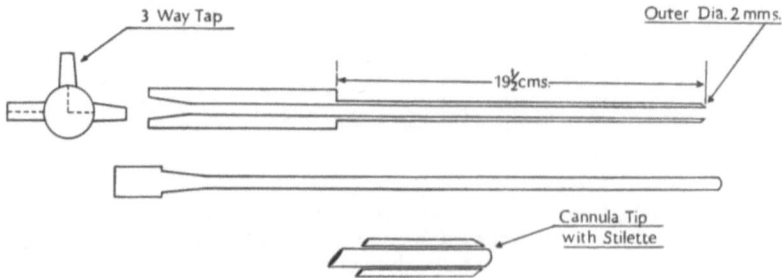

NOT TO SCALE

Fig. 1. The stereotaxic biopsy cannula is illustrated and its mode of use
is given in the text

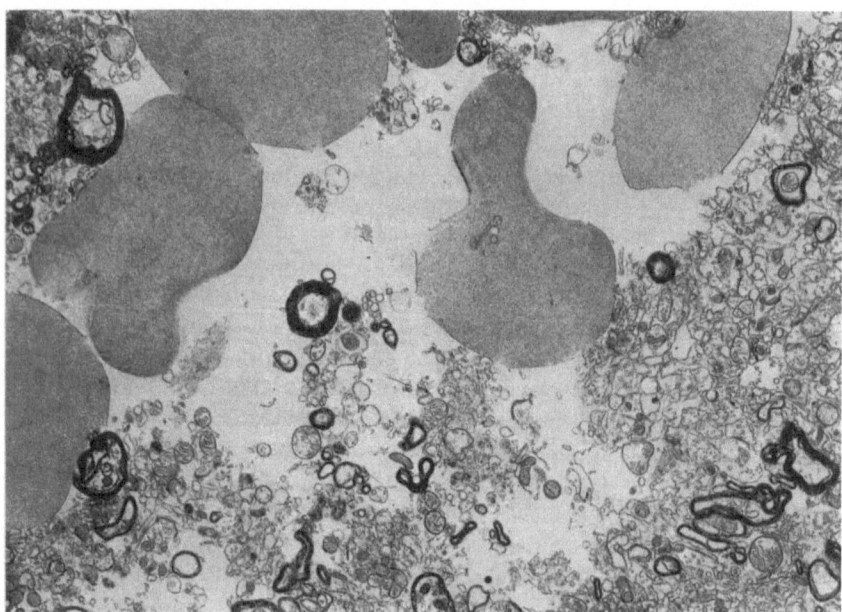

Fig. 2. An electron micrograph of monkey ventralis lateralis nucleus obtained by the stereotaxic biopsy cannula illustrated in Fig. 1. Note the
localized destruction of tissue around the extravasated red blood corpuscles.
× 7,000

scope level of examination. Biopsies were taken by this stereotaxic apparatus from the ventralis lateralis nucleus of the thalamus, fixed in glutaraldehyde with post osmication and embedded in araldite. Silver sections were directly floated onto grids without a supporting membrane and stained with uranyl acetate and lead citrate. A few minute and

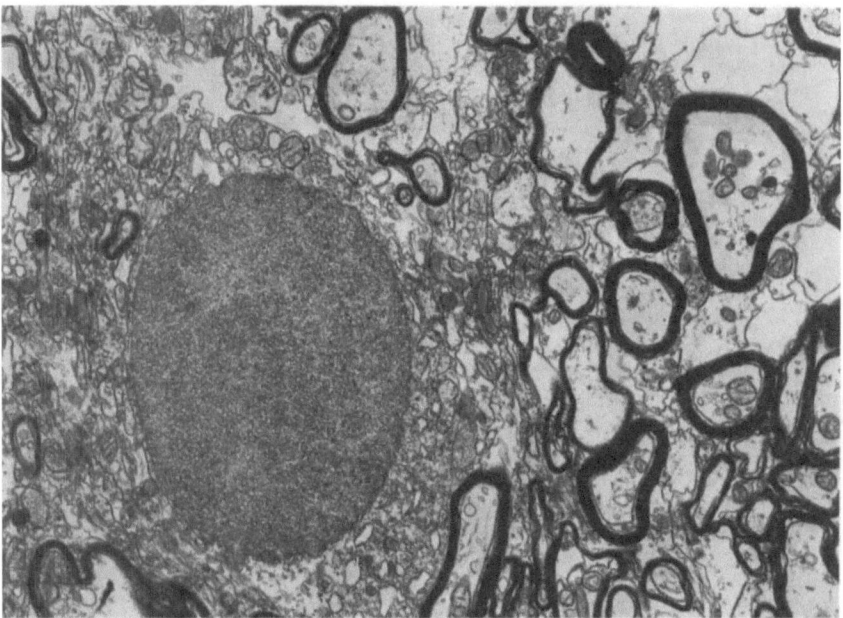

Fig. 3. Similar to Fig. 2. This micrograph is from an area near to that of Fig. 2. The cellular and myelin structure is adequately well preserved and intact. However, a few empty membranous profiles are present at the right side of the micrograph and are probably artifactual consequent upon the surgical method. × 17,500

scattered haemorrhagic lesions were found and even where they comprised only a few extravasated blood corpuscles slight disruption of tissue in their immediate vicinity was always evident. However, fixation and preservation of structure was quite adequate for electron microscopy in most areas. Artifacts induced by the method are shown in Figs. 2–5.

The use of this instrument will be illustrated briefly by a man of 60 years of ago who suffered from porphyria cutanea tarda associated with neurological features. In 1966 the patient complained of scalp ulceration which improved with topical steroids only to recur with associated alopecia. At that time there was found hepatomegaly and alcohol intake was always very moderate. In 1967 the patient started to develop tremor of hands and head which were progressive and almost completely disabled the patient. He was referred to the Department of Neurology, Royal Victoria Infirmary, Newcastle upon Tyne under the care of Dr. Peter Hudgson for investigation. The liver was somewhat hard and enlarged and a compound tremor was present in both upper limbs with Parkinsonian, flapping and

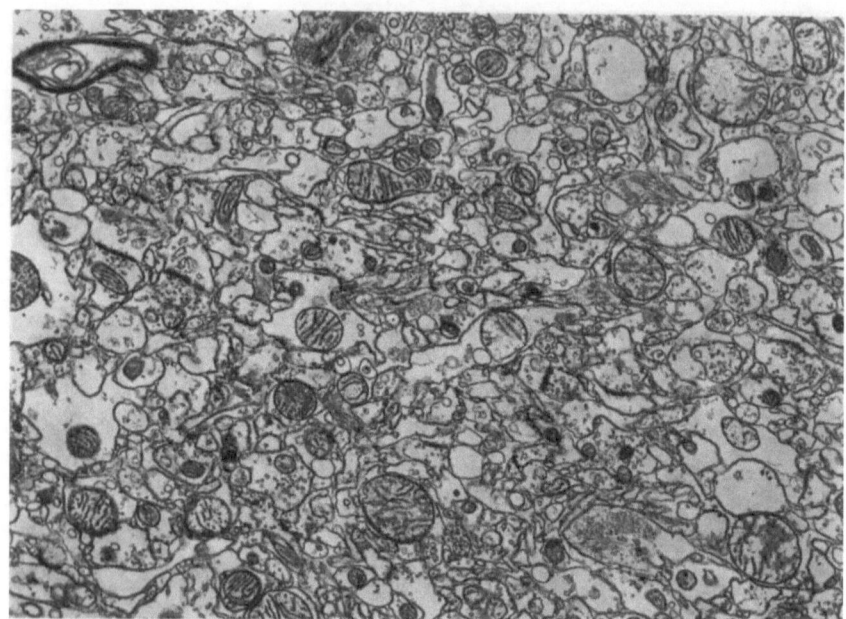

Fig. 4. Similar to Fig. 2. The neuropil is well preserved showing dendrites, synaptic complexes and glial processes. An occasional rather empty membranous profile is present and may be artifactual consequent upon the surgical method. × 20,000

intention elements together with persistent haed nodding and torticollis. It was first thought before investigation that this patient had cirrhosis of the liver with portasystemic encephalopathy but this was not confirmed and a diagnosis of porphyria cutanea tarda was made which was associated with a remarkably high urinary uroporphyrin excretion of 267 µg/l. As was expected a high serum iron was also found and histology of a liver biopsy showed hepatic siderosis.

On 17th June, 1971, a stereotactic lesion was made in the left VL thalamic nucleus and a right VL lesion was made on 18th May, 1972; very considerable improvement ensued. On each occasion a biopsy was taken and prepared for electron microscopy. It was thought possible that the neurological symptomatology was due to a similar cerebral pathology to that found in acute intermittent porphyria which is essentially a demyelinating lesion,

often perivascular and commonly is associated with neuronal chromato-
lytic change (Gibson and Goldberg 1956, Goldberg and Rimington 1962,
Smith and Whittaker 1963). The findings of the present case based upon
electron microscopy, add support to the suggestion made here that the
neurological manifestations which rarely occur in porphyria cutanea tarda
are similar in nature to those of acute intermittent porphyria. Demyelina-

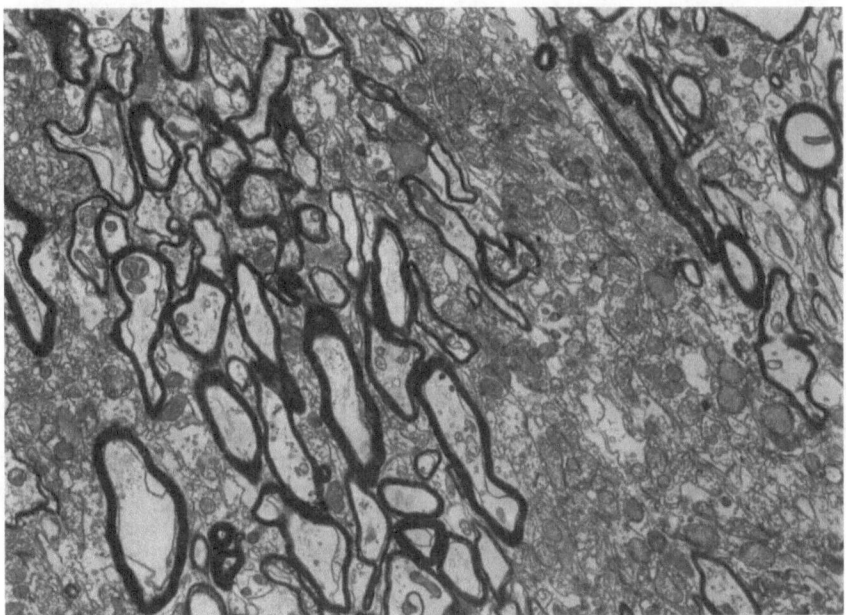

Fig. 5. Similar to Fig. 2. Satisfactory preservation of nerve fibres and
neuropil is present. × 10,500

tion of axons was evident (Fig. 6), pronounced glial proliferation was present
with the astrocytic processes densely filled with fibrillar material and much
lipid and lipofuscin was to be seen. Of particular interest was the finding
of dense perivascular intertwining fibres in 1 μ thick araldite sections
stained by toluidine blue when examined by the light microscope. Electron
microscopy showed these fibres to be formed of fibrils of 1000 Å diameter
which themselves are comprised of filaments 50 Å diameter but without
definite periodicity. Final identification of this material has not been
achieved. The pathological findings will be published in detail elsewhere.

Conclusions

A simple method of obtaining stereotaxic biopsies from the human
brain has been described. The biopsies are suitable for electron microscopy and a few artifacts induced by the method have been illustrated

with material obtained by the instrument from the monkey ventralis lateralis nucleus of the thalamus.

From the clinical point of view the use of the instrument is illustrated by two thalamic ventralis lateralis biopsies obtained from a case of porphyria cutanea tarda complicated by additional neurological features

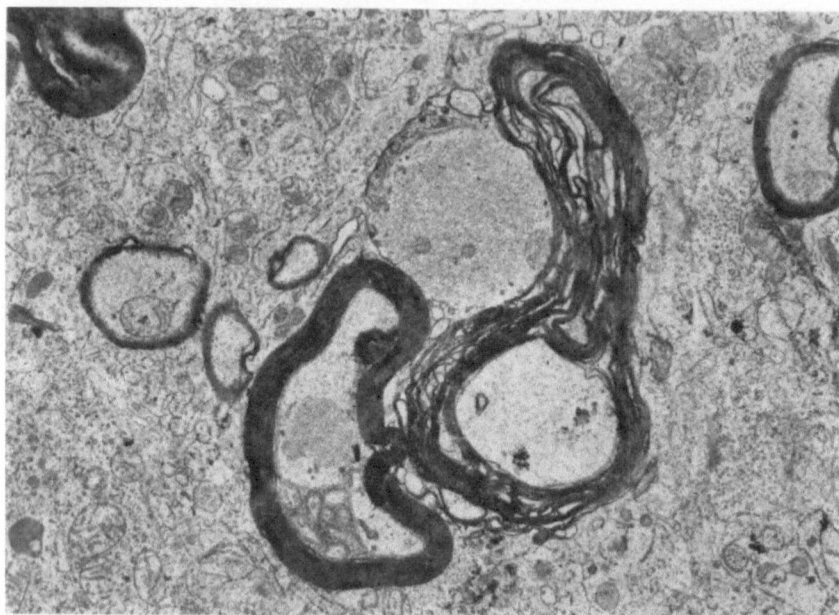

Fig. 6. An electron micrograph from the case of porphyria cutanea tarda showing a nerve fibre with myelin disintegration and adjacent on the left a demyelinated axon filled with neurofilaments. Myelin lamella reduplication and folding is present within the other nearby nerve fibre. × 20,000

which included a bilateral compound tremor of both upper limbs. Electron microscopy of these biopsies showed prominent demyelination of axons, gliosis, lipid accumulations and unusual perivascular fibrils of a type not yet identified with certainty. It is suggested that the cerebral symptoms which may occur in porphyria cutanea tarda are similar to those of acute intermittent porphyria.

Acknowledgements

We acknowledge gratefully the assistance of Dr. B. Odoriz and Dr. P. Martin-Rodriguez for their help in designing the biopsy cannula, surgery and experimental procedures.

We also wish to acknowledge the valuable technical assistance of Mr. M. Taylor and Mr. B. Pugh who were responsible for the preparation of material for electron microscopy and photography.

References

1. Gibson, J. B., Goldberg, A. (1956), The neuropathology of acute porphyria. J. Path. Bact. *71*, 495—509.
2. Goldberg, A., Rimington, C. (1962), Diseases of porphyrin metabolism.
   Springfield, Ill.: Ch. C Thomas.
3. Kalyanaraman, S., Gillingham, F. J. (1964), Stereotaxic biopsy. J.
   Neurosurg. *21*, 854—858.
4. Smith, W. T., Whittaker, S. R. F. (1963), Diffuse degeneration of white
   matter resembling so-called Binswanger's disease and symmetrical
   necrosis of the globus pallidus associated with acute porphyria and cerebral atherosclerosis. J. Clin. Path. *16*, 419—422.

Authors' address: Dr. J. Hankinson, Newcastle General Hospital,
Newcastle upon Tyne, England.

Acta Neurochirurgica, Suppl. 21, 235—243 (1974)
© by Springer-Verlag 1974

Montreal Neurological Institute and Hospital, Canada

Computer Display of Stereotaxic Brain Maps and Probe Tracts

G. Bertrand, A. Olivier, and C. J. Thompson

With 7 Figures

Sooner or later, neurosurgeons engaged in stereotaxic surgery wish to plot on some type of brain atlas the position of their probe tracts or their therapeutic lesions. This is made difficult by the fact that the patient's brain usually differs from the "standard" atlas brain in its dimensions and one wonders, then, how to match the two. Should one align the anterior commissures, the posterior commissures, the foramina of Monro, the mid commissural points, etc.? Should one use only proportionate measurements? Or use different atlases for brains of different sizes?

Another difficulty arises because probe tracts are usually oblique to at least two of the three stereotaxic planes and, with many techniques, to all three planes. The problem is compounded by the use of side-protruding electrodes capable of exploring along oblique or curved tracts in any direction around the axis of the probe. Even if explorations are deliberately restricted to tracts parallel to one of the planes, the sagittal plane, for instance, these tracts will usually be oblique to the other two planes and it may be difficult to accurately visualize the position of the probe or the lateral extent of the lesion against coronal or horizontal maps.

These are well recognized problems and a number of ingenious devices have been used to obviate them (Bell 1966, Dawson et al. 1968, Riechert and Mundinger 1959).

The task of transposing stereotaxic probe angles and coordinates to brain atlas coordinates is a fairly simple mathematical operation, ideally suited to computerization. Bates and Brewer (1969), Peluso and Gybels (1969, 1970) have published methods to calculate the coordinates of single or side-electrode positions using computerized tables.

The difficulties arising from morphological and dimensional differences have been tackled in a variety of ways. Delmas and Pertuiset (1959) have codified the location of deep cerebral nuclei in relation to

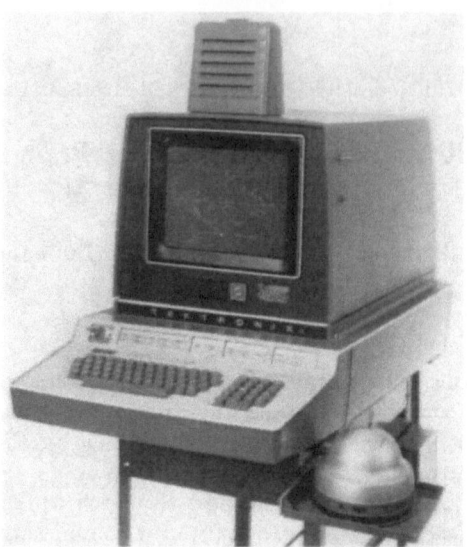

Fig. 1. Tektronix T-4002 "Computer Graphics Terminal". To the right of keyboard, "Joystick", type 015-1075-00, controlling movable crosshairs on screen

ANSWER THE FOLLOWING QUESTIONS:::::::: BY TYPING DISTANCES IN MM, ANGLES IN DEGREES

■■■■■ MAPUNITS VERSION 26/8/71 ■■■■■

WHAT IS THE DISTANCE BETWEEN ANTERIOR AND POSTERIOR COMMISSURES (23) 2 4 . 5

WHAT IS THE HEIGHT OF THE THALAMUS (19.5) 1 8 . 7

WHAT IS THE WIDTH OF THE THIRD VENTRICLE (2) 3 . 2

WHAT IS THE SKEW ANGLE OF THE FRAME (NEGATIVE IF BACK IS LOWER THAN FRONT) 2 5

WHAT IS THE A-P APPROACH ANGLE (NEGATIVE IF FROM BACK) 2 3

WHAT IS THE LATERAL ANGLE OF THE PROBE ON THE MOVING ARC 1 1

IDENTIFY TARGET BY TYPING DISTANCE FROM MIDLINE ON NORMAL SCALE MAP:: THEN

POINT TO TARGET WITH JOYSTICK AND TYPE "T" 1 2 . 7

Fig. 2. Questionnaire as displayed on viewing screen. "Standard" brain dimensions in parentheses. Individual case dimensions and angles appear in larger type (arbitrarily chosen in this example)

cranial measurements. Talairach et al. (1957) use a proportionate system or coordinates subdividing the thalamus and surrounding structures in various geometric "zones de repérage". Other homothetic transformations of the brain maps have been achieved by the use of optical devices (Riechert and Mundinger 1959) or by mathematical coefficients (Riechert and Mundinger 1959, Spiegel and Wycis 1952). More complex transformations have been mapped by means of analogue field plotters (Barcia-Salorio 1969).

The availability of a Digital Equipment Corporation P.D.P. 12 computer near our operating theatre at the Montreal Neurological Institute has led us to explore the possibility of obtaining a computerized graphic display of stereotaxic brain maps and probe tracts.

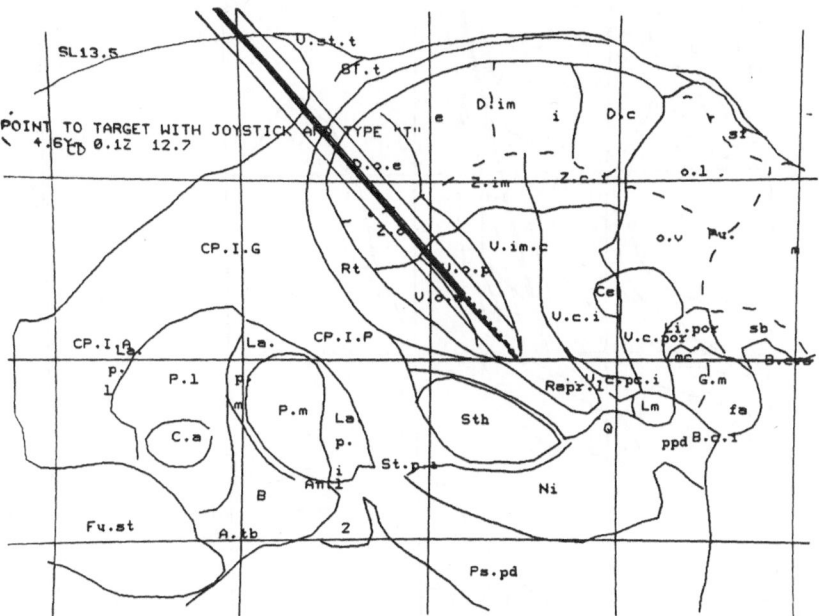

Fig. 3. Photograph of screen display of sagittal section SL 13.5 showing probe on target. Dotted portion of probe lies medial to the section

Suitable programs were written by one of us (C. J. Thompson) to encode on the computer's disk memory 48 of the stereotaxic brain maps from the Schaltenbrand and Bailey atlas. For convenience, a few of the extremely anterior and posterior maps were deleted and some of the maps were trimmed along the edges to include only structures visible on each of the three planes represented, the nomenclature used by Hassler (1959) was also included but was slightly modified, all labels being written horizontally and some shortened.

Transformation of the brain map line drawings to digital data, as stored in the computer memory, was accomplished by tracing enlarged photographs of the transparent line drawings of the Atlas with the

mechanical pen of an analogue X. Y. plotter. The voltages across the
X and Y potentiometers from any given point of the map being trans-
lated into their corresponding digital value by the analogue to digital
converter of the computer.

The drawings obtained could then be displayed on the viewing screen
of a Tektronix type 4002 "Computer Graphics Terminal" and labelled,
using the typewriter keyboard which is part of the terminal. This

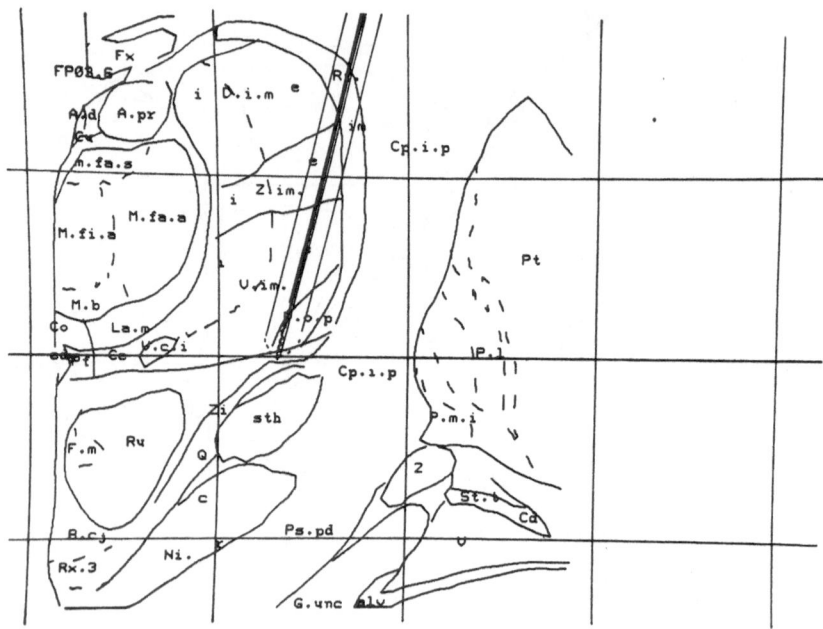

Fig. 4. Same probe position as in Fig. 3, viewed against frontal
section F. P. 3.6 (F. P. 3.5 in S and B Atlas)

terminal and the attached Tektronix type 4901 "Interactive Graphics
Unit and Joystick" type 015-1075-00 are the only part of the instrument
which need to be brought to the operating room (Fig. 1). The computer
itself, its disk memory and the other apparatus can be left in another
part of the building and are connected to the terminal by a small cable.

Once the program is loaded in the computer, a display on the viewing
screen lists the various maps available in the sagittal, frontal and horizontal planes. It also asks a number of questions, the answers to which
are readily available from simple measurements on the stereotaxic
ventriculogram: the distance between the commissures, the height of
the thalamus above the intercommissural plane, if visible; the width

of the third ventricle (Fig. 2). Answers to these questions are simply typed on the terminal keyboard. They are used to compress or expand the corresponding dimensions of the map to match the individual patient's brain, at least as far as the X-ray landmarks are concerned.

For the moment, we are not using any compression or stretching in the Z axis (medio-lateral direction) but only shift the map laterally or medially according to the width of the third ventricle. The brains used

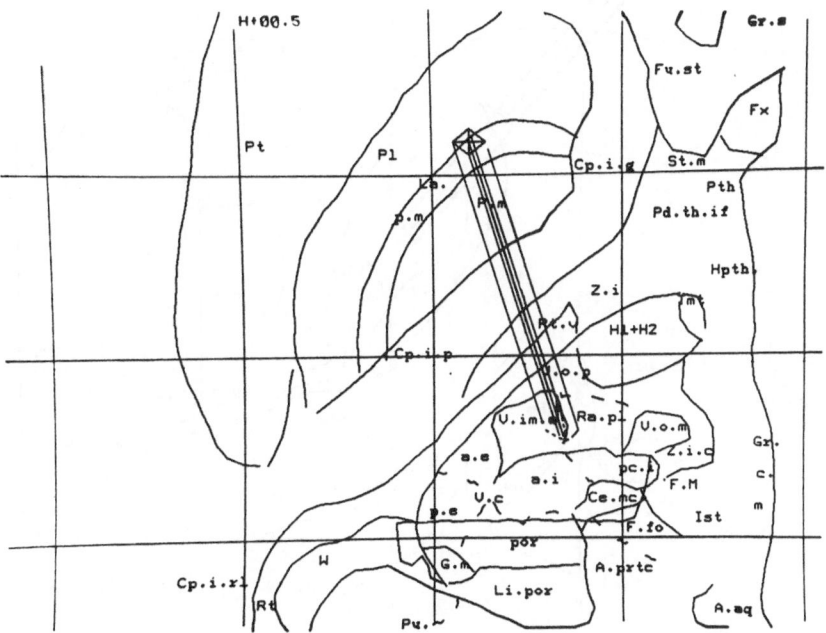

Fig. 5. Same probe projected against horizontal section H. D. 0.5

for the Atlas, particularly for the frontal section, being narrower than average, methods are now being studied to expand the maps in accordance to other available measurements.

The computer, at this stage, can display any of the available maps corrected to fit the patient's ventricular landmarks. By moving the "Joystick", one can move "cross hairs" on the viewing screen and point to any structure at will. By pressing the appropriate key, one can then obtain views in another plane corresponding to the level indicated by the horizontal or the vertical line of the "cross hairs". The computer will automatically select, scale and display the map nearest to the desired level. It also compensates for the fact that, in the Schaltenbrand and

Bailey Atlas, the "horizontal" maps are not parallel to the intercommissural plane but are angled 8° on it.

Another set of questions concerns the angles between the intercommissural plane and the horizontal base of the instrument (we use a
modified Leksell instrument, Bertrand et al. 1969) and angles of introduction of the probe in relation to the midsagittal plane and the horizontal base of the instrument (Figs. 2).

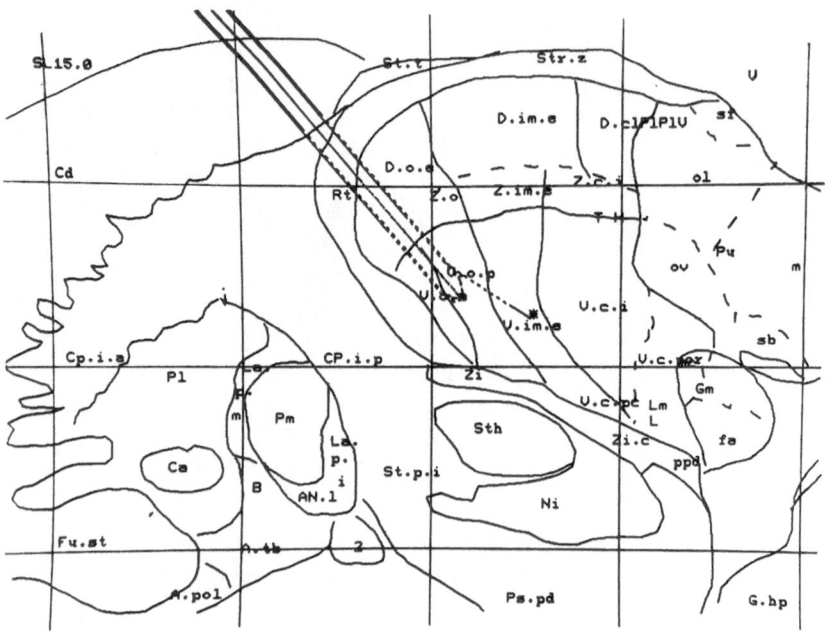

Fig. 6. Projection of a curved side-electrode against sagittal plane S. L. 15.0.
Most of the probe shaft lies medial to the plane shown but the tip of the
side-electrode, being directed laterally and back, emerges from the plane
in the last 2 mm

By indicating the distance from the midline at which, on an average
brain, one would like to make the lesion, the sagittal section nearest
to this plane is displayed. If one then points on this map, with the
"Joystick" cross-hairs, to the location of the target as selected on the
ventriculogram, the image of a straight probe, suitably directed to
target, appears (Fig. 3). That portion of the probe which lies beyond
the displayed plane appears as a dotted outline.

Any plane at right angles to the one displayed or parallel to it can
then be demonstrated by moving the "Joystick" cross-hairs and typing

the appropriate key (H. for horizontal, F. for frontal) and the probe will be displayed as seen in this new projection (Figs. 4 and 5).

The use of side-protruding electrodes or leucotomes calls for another set of questions on the screen concerning the type of probe used (serial number), the distance at which it is introduced above or below target, the direction around the axis of the probe in which the side-electrode is extended and how much of the side-electrode (or leucotome) is out of

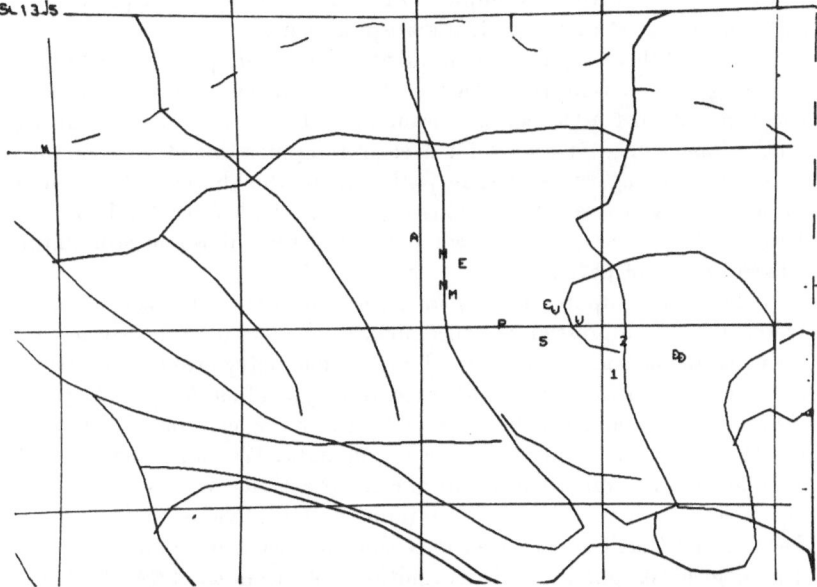

Fig. 7. Enlarged portion of sagittal section S. L. 13.5 showing points where various responses were obtained.   Grid lines now indicate 5 mm and do not coincide with stereotaxic coordinates

the shaft. The chosen probe can then be shown on the "scaled" sagittal, frontal or horizontal maps, in the same way as for a straight probe (Fig. 6).

As the electrodes are advanced, different patterns of recorded cellular activity or responses to stimulation are encountered. It is useful to keep track of these phenomena and, as they are observed, each can be given a code letter and inscribed on computer tape or disk memory. At the end of the exploration or later, this data can be recalled and shown on maps from which, for clarity, labels have been omitted. Data from many patients can then be pooled and compared in various combinations and displayed according to type of responses or to show "slices" of varying thickness in which all types of responses encountered are shown.

Since areas of interest tend to be small and symbols closely packed, it is possible to enlarge a particular area of the map to occupy the entire screen and still retain accurate proportions and be able to shift from one plane to the other at will (Fig. 7).

Polaroid photographs of the screen can be taken at any time for permanent record but anything displayed on the screen can also be drawn on paper with a "Complot D.P. 1-N 2" incremental plotter and then becomes part of the patient's hospital chart.

This use of the computer is a useful adjunct to our operative technique, providing for constant visualization, during surgery, of our electrode or leucotome against a stereotaxic brain atlas better adapted to our patient's dimensions. It allows for a clearer appreciation of the structures encountered along the electrode path and of the shape and extent of the lesion in the three dimensions of space. It also greatly facilitates the retrospective analysis and comparison of recording and stimulation data in groups of patients.

So far, our computer is only an electronic brain atlas which can be stretched or compressed to accomodate to patient's measurements. The instrument has no difficulty solving trigonometry problems involving multiple angles and is ideally adapted to a type of surgery dealing with tridimensional geometry but we feel that more can be asked of it, particularly in the analysis of recording data. We hope that it may be taught to discriminate patterns of cellular activity or variations in cell population density which are not immediately obvious to the human observer and that the computer may thus help to achieve more accurate physiological mapping (and recognition) of deep cerebral structures and more precise surgery.

References

1. Barcia-Salorio, J. L., Martinez Corrillo, J. A. (1969), Calculation of the target point by means of an analogue field plotter, in: Third Symposium on Parkinson's Disease (F. J. Gillingham and I. M. L. Donaldson, eds.), pp. 223—232. London: E. & S. Livingstone.
2. Bates, J. A. V., Brewer, A. (1968), Geometric aspects of stereotaxic surgery. London: (unpublished manuscript).
3. Bell, D. (1966), A stereotaxic principle using a non mathematical three dimensional approach. Investigative Radiology 1 (cited by Dawson, B. H., et al.).
4. Bertrand, G., Jasper, H., Wong, A., Mathews, G. (1969), Microelectrode recording during stereotaxic surgery. Clin. Neurosurg. 16, 328—355.
5. Dawson, B. H., Derrin, E., Heywood, O. B. (1968/69), Bio-engineering approach to stereotaxic surgery of the brain. Proc. Instn. Mech. Engrs. 183, 281—297.

6. Delmas, A., Pertuiset, B. (1959), Topométrie cranio-encéphalique chez l'homme. Paris: Masson. Springfield, Ill.: Ch. C Thomas.
7. Hassler, R. (1959), Anatomy of the thalamus. In: Introduction to Stereotaxy with an atlas of the human brain, vol. 1, pp. 230—290 (Schaltenbrand, G., and Bailey, P., eds.). Stuttgart: G. Thieme.
8. Peluso, F., Gybels, J. (1969), Computer calculation of two-target trajectory with "centre of area target" stereotaxic equipment. Acta neurochir. *21*, 173—180.
9. — — (1970), Calculation of position of electrode point during penetration in human brain. Confin. Neurol. *32*, 213—218.
10. — — Computer calculation of the position of the side-protruding electrode tip during penetration in human brain (unpublished manuscript).
11. Riechert, T., Mundinger, F. (1959), Stereotaxic instruments. In: Introduction to stereotaxy with an atlas of the human brain. Vol. 1, pp. 437—471 (Schaltenbrand, B., and Bailey, P., eds.). Stuttgart: G. Thieme.
12. Spiegel, E. A., Wycis, H. T. (1952), Stereocencephalotomy (thalamotomy and related procedures). Part I: Methods and stereotaxic atlas of the human brain. New York: Grune and Stratton.
13. Talairach, J., David, M., Tournoux, P., Corredor, H., Kvasina, T. (1957), Atlas d'anatomie stéréotaxique. Repérage radiologique indirect des noyaux gris centraux des régions mésencéphalo-sous-optique et hypothalamique de l'homme. Paris: Masson.

Authors' address: G. Bertrand, M.D., 3801 University Street, Montreal 112, P. Que., Canada.

Acta Neurochirurgica, Suppl. 21, 245—252 (1974)
© by Springer-Verlag 1974

Department of Mechanical Engineering, University of Salford,
and Department of Neurological Surgery,
Salford Royal Hospital, Salford, England

The Use of a Small Digital Computer
for Stereotactic Surgery

E. Dervin, O. B. Heywood, T. R. Crossley, and B. H. Dawson

With 8 Figures

Introduction

There are many stereotactic systems available for the direction of
fine surgical instruments into the deeply situated nuclei of the brain.
In some of these techniques the location of the target and the calculation
of the corresponding settings on the stereotactic frame are determined
by approximate two-dimensional solutions. In others, careful alignment
of the axes of the stereotactic frame with the mid-plane of the brain
can simplify complicated three-dimensional mathematics to two-
dimensional problems. The use of digital computers to calculate accurate
frame settings to reach chosen targets in the brain is an obvious but
expensive way of eliminating the need for time consuming alignment
procedures.

Experimental work in the University of Salford, the Salford Royal
Hospital and Walton Hospital, Liverpool, has shown that inexpensive
and portable desk-top computers can be programmed for use with any
stereotactic method which employs a reference system of rectangular
cartesian co-ordinates.

Alignment Problems

In a stereotactic operation using a rectangular co-ordinate frame,
for example, the Leksell[1] (1949) device, great care is usually taken to
place the frame symmetrically on the patient's skull so that the mid-
sagittal plane of the patient's ventricular system and the mid-plane
of the reference frame are in alignment. Simple calculations from the

radiographic data can then be made to obtain frame settings to guide the electrode to a chosen target in the brain.

Inadvertent misalignment of the co-ordinate frame may make calculation of the frame settings difficult and tedious because the associated geometrical problems are of a complex three-dimensional nature. Similar difficulties also occur when there is pathological asymmetry of the patient's ventricular system even if the frame is aligned correctly with the skull.

The effects of frame misalignment, Figs. 1 and 2, may be classified as follows:

a) Rotation of the brain about an axis parallel to the horizontal lateral (Z) axis of the frame, Fig. 1 (a).

b) Rotation of the brain about an axis parallel to the horizontal antero-posterior (X) axis of the frame, Fig. 1 (b).

c) Rotation of the brain about an axis parallel to the vertical (Y) axis of the frame, Fig. 1 (c).

d) Linear displacements of the brain relative to the axes of the frame but maintaining parallelism of the brain axes with the frame axes, Fig. 2. Each of these effects may occur with any combination of the other three.

Linear displacements are readily recognized on radiographs and easily allowed for in the calculation of the frame settings. Unfortunately, these linear displacements rarely occur without associated rotational displacements.

The Computer Technique

The mathematical problem is to establish the position and orientation of the ventricular reference structures of the brain relative to the axes of the stereotactic reference frame from radiographic input data. The computer can then be programmed to give frame settings for any chosen target in the brain.

In the Salford technique the ventricular reference structures are based on the Schaltenbrand and Bailey atlas (anterior commissure, posterior commissure and mid-sagittal plane), or the Andrew and Watkins atlas (Foramen of Munro, posterior commissure and mid-sagittal plane). Fig. 3 shows the appropriate axes of the brain for each system.

Using the Leksell reference frame as an example, the radiographic input data required for the computer consists of eleven readings which are illustrated in Fig. 4. Eight of the readings are taken from the lateral radiograph and three readings are taken from the antero-posterior radiograph. The paths taken by the X-rays through the ventricular reference points (ac and pc) are shown. These two "commissural rays" diverge from the X-ray source and intersect the left-hand plane of the

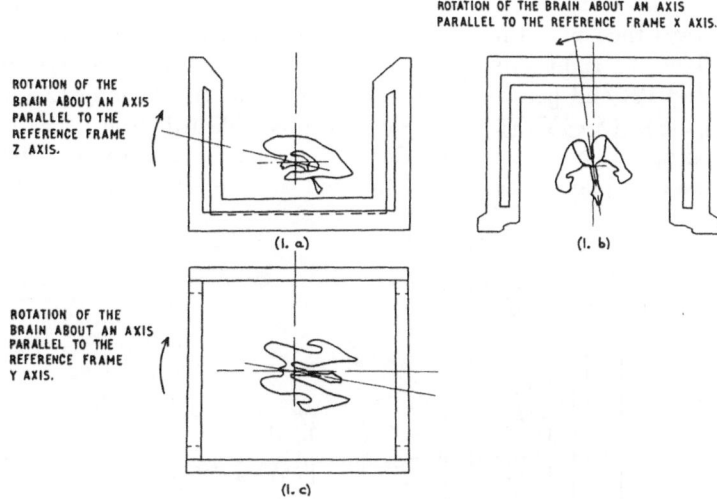

Fig. 1. Rotational displacements between brain axes and reference frame
axes

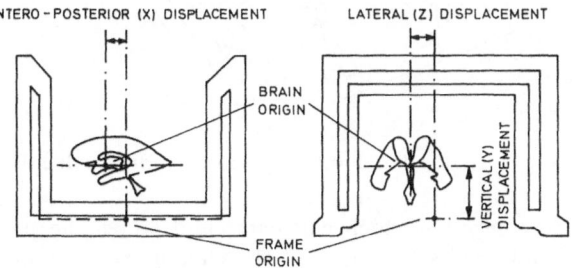

Fig. 2. Linear displacements between brain axes and reference frame axes

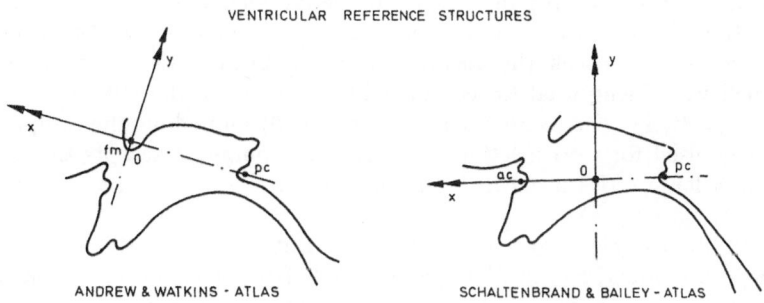

Fig. 3. Alternative systems of brain axes

co-ordinate frame at two points which are represented by AL and PL. The rays then pass through the anterior and posterior commissures to intersect the right-hand plane of the co-ordinate frame at two points AR and PR and pass through to the film. The co-ordinates $(X_{AL}Y_{AL})$, $(X_{PL}Y_{PL})$, $(X_{AR}Y_{AR})$, $(X_{PR}Y_{PR})$ are established from the lateral radiograph. The antero-posterior radiograph is used to establish the mid-sagittal plane data Z_{DAS}, Z_{DPS} and α. The eleven co-ordinates are

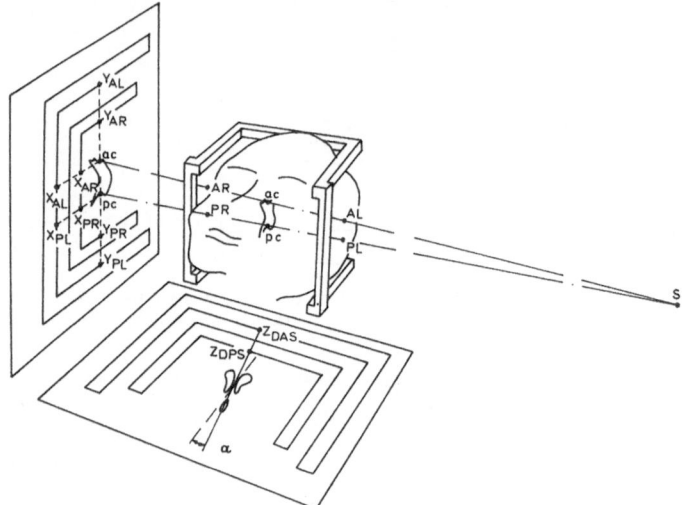

Fig. 4. Lateral and antero-posterior radiographic data

fed into the computer which calculates and stores the position of the brain axes and awaits the input of the chosen target co-ordinates from a brain atlas.

In Salford the analysis by computer was originally developed by Dawson et al.[2] (1970) for the retrospective analysis of the lesion site positions for a series of stereotactic procedures for the relief of Parkinsonism and to check the accuracy of mechanical analogue techniques which were being used for computation, Dawson et al.[3] (1969).

A portion of the computer print-out (Fig. 5) shows how the computer can be used for retrospective analysis. The computer accepts the data from a large series of patients and prints out the results in any desired format.

In the sample shown the computer prints out the patient's name, hospital number, length of ac/pc line (or FM/pc) the co-ordinates of the origin of the patient's brain and the co-ordinates of the lesion site for the given frame settings.

STEREOTAXIS

NUMBER	LENGTH		X	Y	Z
(21) 8245	+26.6204	ORIGIN	+0.2587	+47.5236	+4.2447
		FRAME	-4.0000	+48.0000	+15.0000
* Wiles	(R)	BRAIN	-4.4374	+0.6628	+10.6728
(22) 8237	+25.3034	ORIGIN	-10.2583	+46.5195	+3.4430
		FRAME	-15.0000	+46.0000	+15.0000
Berry	(R)	BRAIN	-4.5544	+1.1857	+11.5932
(23) 8335	+18.0934	ORIGIN	-8.9102	+38.8242	+7.8536
		FRAME	-13.0000	+39.0000	+17.0000
Raby	(R)	BRAIN	-4.4015	-0.5521	+9.0214
(24) 8245	+26.2009	ORIGIN	-3.8151	+48.9532	-8.4259
		FRAME	-9.0000	+50.0000	+2.0000
* Wiles	(2R)	BRAIN	-5.0116	-0.0660	+10.5621
(25) 8518	+25.4589	ORIGIN	-13.4690	+45.3950	-19.3726
		FRAME	-18.0000	+45.0000	-10.0000
Holmes	(R)	BRAIN	-4.1167	+2.1032	+9.3360
(26) 8481	+20.5244	ORIGIN	+3.2500	+45.5000	+0.0000
		FRAME	+2.0000	+46.0000	-8.0000
Bray	(L)	BRAIN	-1.2242	+0.5603	-8.0000
(27) 8558	+25.0050	ORIGIN	-5.5000	+46.2500	+0.0000
		FRAME	-10.0000	+46.0000	-12.0000
Melling	(L)	BRAIN	-4.5041	-0.1600	-12.0000
(28) 8683	+24.3447	ORIGIN	-2.9882	+43.0241	-3.2656
		FRAME	-7.0000	+48.0000	+10.0000
Whittle	(R)	BRAIN	-1.9763	+5.3680	+13.5687
(29) 8345	+22.8555	ORIGIN	+3.2583	+39.2417	+3.0000
		FRAME	+0.0000	+47.0000	+15.0000
Jones	(R)	BRAIN	-2.0258	+8.1673	+12.0000
(30) 8145	+25.0114	ORIGIN	-8.4806	+50.7222	-3.3521
		FRAME	-12.0000	+55.0000	-15.0000
Ashworth	(L)	BRAIN	-3.1216	+4.8142	-11.5515

Fig. 5. Sample of computer print out in a series of patients

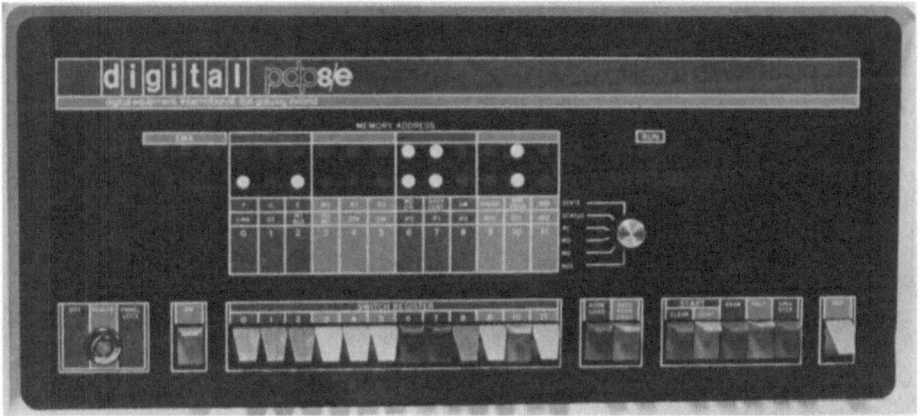

Fig. 6. Front panel of Digital PDP 8e desk top calculator

For the purposes of this analysis the data was fed via a tele-type link to the central computer in the University of Salford. During the course of these analyses, irritating failures and delays occurred due to faults in the link to the computer.

This lack of reliability of the long range tele-type link to a large central computer system discouraged its use in the operating suite as a

```
*GO

NO:593G
XAL:7 YAL:51 XAR:10 YAR:57
XPL:-17 YPL:46 XPR:-22 YPR:48
ZDAS:-4 ZDPS:-6
ALPHA:-3

ORIGIN
X0=-    5.4925    Y0=    50.4670    Z0=-    1.4694

AC/PC=    28.7905

ATLAS
ZB:-8
XB:-12 YB:5
XB(M)=-   15.0211

FRAME
X=-   21.1870    Y=    51.2582    Z=-    9.6967


ATLAS
ZB:0

FRAME
X:-22 Y:51 Z:-10

BRAIN ACTUAL
XB=-   15.8719    YB=    4.9625    ZB=-    8.3074
XB(ATLAS)=-   12.6796

NO:0
*
```

Fig. 7. Print out from mini computer, the input data is underlined

primary means of guidance for the surgical team. The alternative of using a digital computer in the operating suite has now become a possibility, even for intermittent use, with the development of the mini-computer industry which has produced small inexpensive reliable units.

Experience in the University of Salford, Salford Royal Hospital and Walton Hospital, Liverpool has shown that the stereotactic calculations can be programmed into a small portable desk-top computer of the type shown in Fig. 6, which can be used either to direct or, alternatively, to track the pathway of an electrode or probe in three dimensions. This small computer has been programmed to calculate and store the position of the brain axes from the input data of radiographic readings and then print out sets of frame co-ordinates for any number of chosen brain targets. In addition, the computer will translate any set of frame settings into brain co-ordinates.

The length of the ac/pc line (or FM/pc) is computed from the radiographic input data and compared to the value in the reference atlas.

Subsequent data for the brain target co-ordinates is automatically proportioned by the computer which will feed back to the surgical team the actual atlas co-ordinates, the modified co-ordinates and the corresponding frame settings.

Fig. 7 shows a sample print out from the small computer. Input data is underlined for clarity.

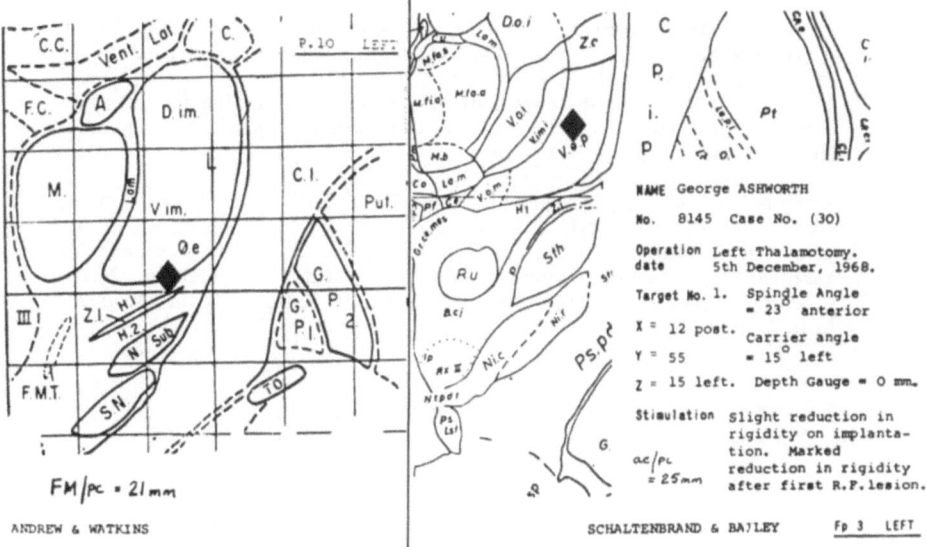

Fig. 8. Corresponding lesion sites mapped on alternative brain atlases

It is also possible to use the computer to map and compare the lesion site positions on alternative systems of brain axes. Fig. 8 illustrates a lesion site for an operation for Parkinson's disease. The lesion has been mapped using both the Andrew and Watkins atlas and the Schaltenbrand and Bailey atlas.

Summary

The advantages in the use of the small computer are:

(i) gives rapid accurate solution to the three-dimensional problems of stereotaxis and overcomes the difficulties when the frame is misaligned;

(ii) any member of the surgical team can be easily trained to use the computer and it is unnecessary to rely on the services of a mathematician or engineer during the operation;

(iii) the computer is in the operating suite, readily available and under the direct control of the surgical team;

(iv) the desk-top computer is relatively inexpensive and because of its portability can be used as a standard piece of computing equipment in other research problems, if it is not wholly occupied by stereotactic procedures.

References

1. Leksell, L. (1949), Stereotactic apparatus for intracerebral surgery. Acta chir. scand. *99*, 229—233.
2. Dawson, B. H., Dervin, E., Heywood, O. B. (1970), Geometrical problems in stereotactic surgery: a three-dimensional analysis for use with computer techniques. J. Biomech. *3*, 175—180.
3. — — — (1969), The development of a mechanical analog for directing and tracking the electrode during stereotaxic operations. Technical Note. J. Neurosurg. *31*, 361—366.

Authors' addresses: E. Dervin, B.Sc (Tech.), Ph.D., C. Eng., M. I. Mech. E., O. B. Heywood, B.Sc (Eng.), C. Eng., M. I. Mech. E., T. R. Crossley, B.Sc (Eng.), Ph.D., C. Eng., A. F. R. Ae. S., Department of Mechanical Engineering, University of Salford, and B. H. Dawson, M.D., F. R. C. S., Department of Neurological Surgery, Salford Royal Hospital, Salford, England.

Acta Neurochirurgica, Suppl. 21, 253—264 (1974)
© by Springer-Verlag 1974

Centro di Terapia Stereotassica "Stella Fossati" and Servizio di Fisica
Sanitaria, Ospedale Maggiore Ca'Granda Milano, Italy

Mathematical Models and Analogic Dosimetry on Phantom in the Interstitial Radiotherapy of Brain Tumours with "Gamma-Med"

G. B. Delzanno, L. Redaelli, and G. Tosi

With 15 Figures

Introduction

In order to employ the "Gamma-Med" apparatus for interstitial radiotherapy of brain tumours, it is primarily necessary to know with maximum accuracy the pattern of the absorbed dose distribution around the source, in the so called "target volume" and also the values of the absorbed dose in the neighbouring tissues and organs, with special regard to the more radiosensitive ones.

In order to achieve this aim it is advisable to use a mathematical model to describe the radiation field around the source and then to verify the results obtained by using suitable instruments, that is performing an analogic dosimetry.

Mathematical Model of Calculus

A. Description of the Radioactive Source

The "Gamma-Med" apparatus consists of a shielded container inside which is a cylindrical source of ^{192}Ir, which can be automatically extracted and inserted in the container itself, to permit introducing the source in the brain via a hollow, flexible plastic cable and a hollow rigid metal guide.

Extraction of the source is automatically performed outside the treatment room. The radioactive source has a length of 16 mm composed of 16 small cylinders, each of which is 1 mm length and 1.8 mm diameter. The source is covered by a thin layer of monel 0.1 mm thick. Moreover, during clinical use, the source is precisely inserted in a stereotactic guide of inox, whose wall is 0.1 mm thick.

The maximum total activity of the sources employed is of the order of 100 curies, while the other physical constants of the source itself, are:

half life   = 74.4 days
mean energy of the gamma radiation   = 360 keV
specific γ-ray constant in water   = 4.59 rad $\cdot$ cm^2/mCi $\cdot$ h

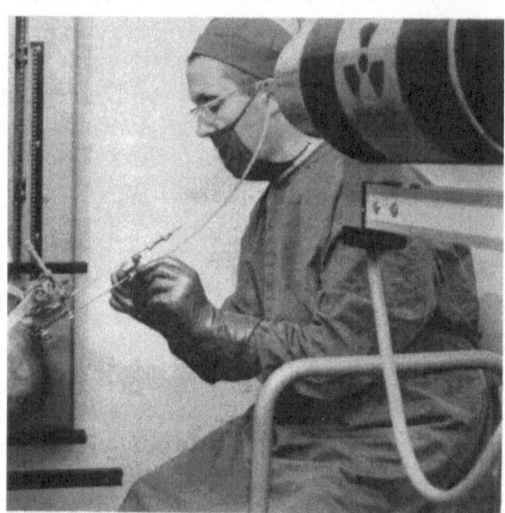

Fig. 1. The use of the "Gamma-Med" apparatus

For computation of the dose, we have taken into account the following assumptions:

1. the linear activity of the source is uniform throughout all the length of the source itself;

2. the decay of the source's activity during the irradiation can be neglected.

In a first approximation, therefore ignoring the self-absorption of the source (due to its thickness), the following formulas for the computation of the dose may be used:

$$D_P = K \cdot \frac{A}{L} \cdot \frac{1}{h} \, (\varphi_1 + \varphi_2)$$

or

$$D_P = K \cdot \frac{A}{L} \cdot \frac{1}{h} \, (\arctan l_1/h + \arctan l_2/h),$$

where:

K is the specific γ-ray constant in water;

A is the total activity of the source, expressed in mCi;

L is the total active length of the source, expressed in cm;

h is the distance, expressed in cm, from the considered point P to the source;

l_1, l_2 are the lengths of the two parts in which the total length L is divided by the projection of the considered point.

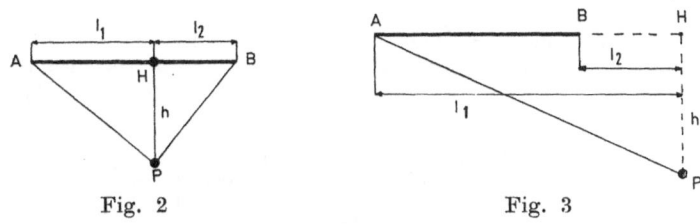

Fig. 2   Fig. 3

Fig. 2. Calculation of the dose in the points of the volume around the source whose projection on the right line containing the source falls inside the source itself.   Self-absorption is not taken into account

Fig. 3. Calculation of the dose in the points of the volume around the source whose projection on the right line containing the source falls outside the source itself.   Self-absorption is not taken into account

This formula, as illustrated in Fig. 2, holds for the calculation of the dose-rate—expressed in rad/h—in the points of the surrounding space, whose projection on the right line containing the source itself falls into the source.

For the points whose projection falls outside the source, the following formula holds (s. Fig. 3):

$$D_P = K \cdot \frac{A}{L} \cdot \frac{1}{h} (\varphi_1 - \varphi_2)$$

or

$$D_P = K \cdot \frac{A}{L} \cdot \frac{1}{h} (\arctan l_1/h - \arctan l_2/h).$$

For the points located on the right line containing the source and, of course, outside the source itself, self-absorption must be taken into account (s. Fig. 4) and this formula holds

$$D_P = K \cdot \frac{A}{L} \int_{h}^{h+1} \frac{1}{x^2} e^{-\mu (x-h)} \, dx$$

where h is the distance between the considered point and the nearest extremity of the source.

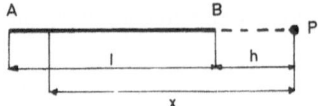

Fig. 4. Calculation of the dose in the points located on the rightline containing the source and outside the source. Self-absorption is taken into account

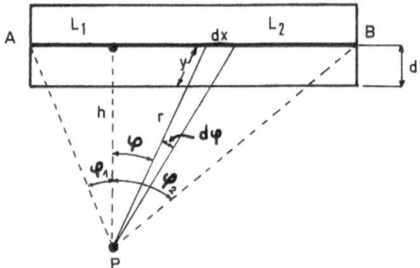

Fig. 5. Calculation of the dose taking into account self-absorption

In order to take self-absorption into account it is possible, with a good approximation, to suppose that all the active material of the source is concentrated on the cylinder's axes and is surrounded by a thickness of absorbing material equal to the radius of the source.

Since self-absorption plays a different role in correspondence of the various energies of ^{192}Ir spectrum, it is necessary to evaluate separately the contribution to the dose of each monochromatic component. After such calculations, one observes that it is possible to obtain the same result in a simpler manner, that is by introducing a suitable average absorption coefficient $\bar{\mu}_a$, depending on the source's geometry.

For the dose calculation it is therefore possible to employ the following formula (s. Fig. 5):

$$D_P = K \cdot \frac{A}{L} \cdot \left\{ \int_{0}^{L_1} \frac{dx}{r^2} e^{-\bar{\mu}_a y} \pm \int_{0}^{L_2} \frac{dx}{r_2} e^{-\bar{\mu}_a y} \right\}$$

or

$$D_P = K \cdot \frac{A}{L} \cdot \left\{ \int\limits_0^{\varphi_1} \frac{e^{\frac{-\bar{\mu}_a d}{\cos \varphi}}}{h} \, d\varphi \pm \int\limits_0^{\varphi_2} \frac{e^{\frac{-\bar{\mu}_a d}{\cos \varphi}}}{h} \right\} d\varphi$$

where:

$\bar{\mu}_a = 3.565 \ cm^{-1}$ is the average linear self-absorption coefficient of the source, and

d is the radius of the source.

In Table 1 are compared the dose values in the symmetry plane perpendicular to the source's axes, obtained without taking and, conversely, taking into account self-absorption. At a distance of 1 cm from the source's axes, the difference is nearly 30%.

Table 1. *Intensity of the Absorbed Dose (Expressed in rad/min for 100 Ci) in Function of the Distance h from the Center of the Source's Axes, in the Plane Perpendicular to the Source in Its Center*

h (mm)	I_1	I_2
2	63387	38848
4	26469	17783
6	14781	10204
8	9385	6581
10	6448	4563
12	4687	3332
14	3541	2531
16	2770	1983
18	2218	1592

I_1 Intensity of the absorbed dose without taking into account self-absorption.
I_2 Intensity of the absorbed dose taking into account self-absorption.

The isodose curves in each plane containing the source are illustrated in Figs. 6 and 7.

From these figures one observes a very marked decrease of the absorbed dose departing from the source: at a distance of 10 mm from the source's axes, the dose is indeed 15% of the dose at 3 mm, while at 20 mm it is only about 5%. Besides, the absorbed dose around the source is very high and of the order of 250% at 1 mm distance.

All this suggests it is impossible to give a sufficient dose on the periphery of relatively extended tumours, that is of tumours of more than 3 cm diameter.

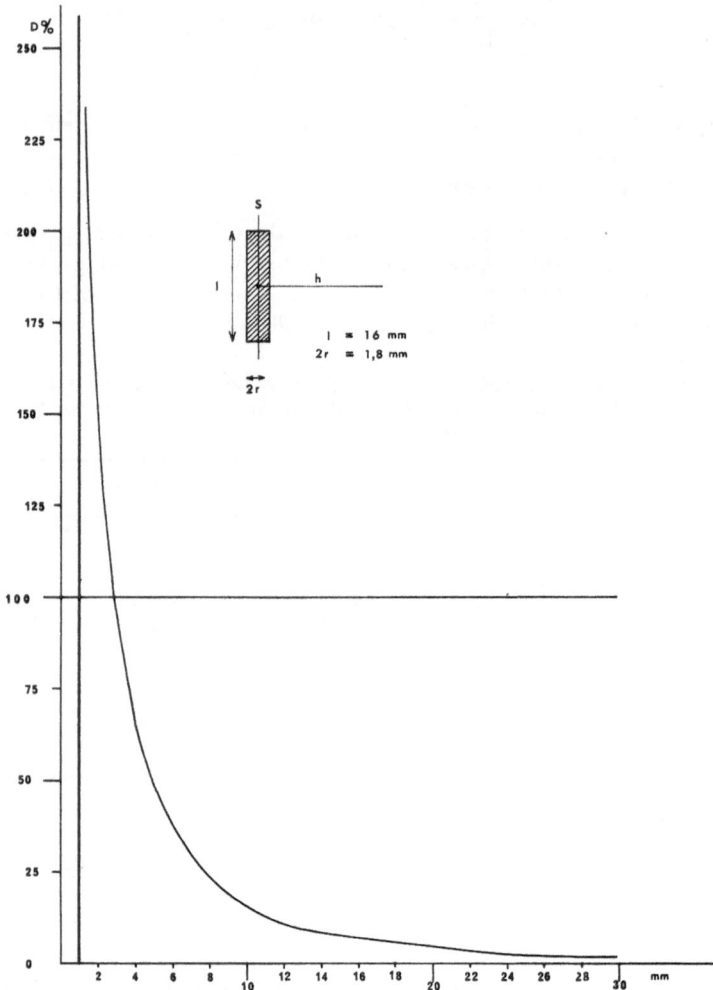

Fig. 6. Trend of the dose in radial direction in a plane perpendicular to
the source in its center

In order to obtain a better dose distribution in target volumes of more than 3 cm diameter, we have therefore studied the possibility of putting the source in more than one position. To determine the isodose curves in these cases, we have employed the principle of super-position,

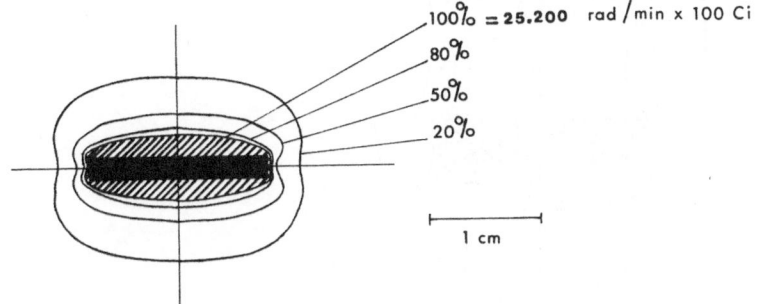

Fig. 7. Isodose curves in the planes containing the source

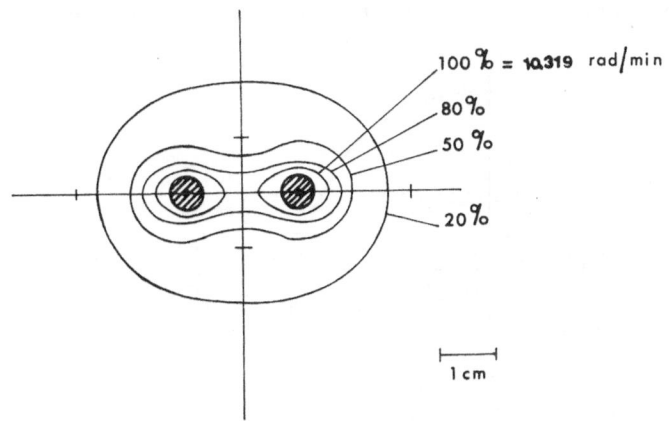

Fig. 8. Source in two parallel positions, at a distance of 15 mm. Isodose curves in the plane containing the two positions

that is: the dose in one point is calculated as the sum of the contribution in the same point from the various positions of the source.

Fig. 8 and Fig. 9 illustrate the dose distribution in the case where the source is placed in two positions parallel to each other at the distance of 15 mm; in Fig. 7 the isodose curves are represented on the plane containing the two positions and in Fig. 9 on the plane perpendicular to the preceding one and passing for the source's center.

In Figs. 10 and 11 are illustrated the isodose curves for a similar case,

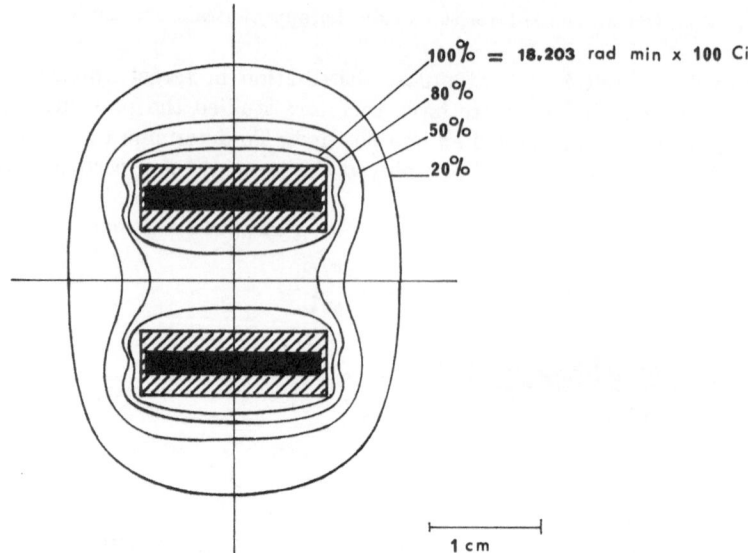

Fig. 9. The same disposition as in Fig. 8. Isodose curves in the plane
perpendicular to the two positions and passing for their centers

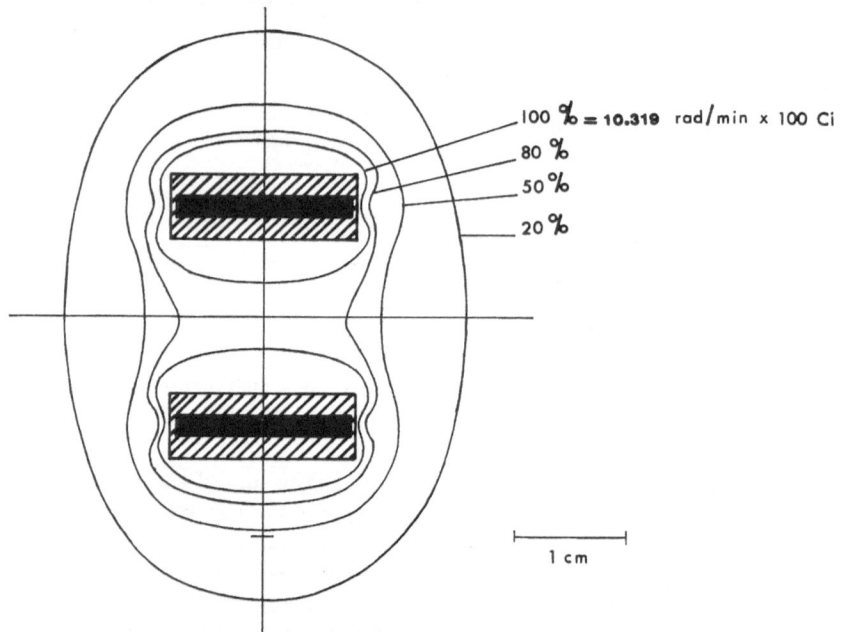

Fig. 10. Source in two parallel positions, at a distance of 20 mm.
Isodose curves in the plane containing the two positions

in which, however, the distance between the two positions of the source is 20 mm.

In Fig. 12 are illustrated—in the case in which the source is placed

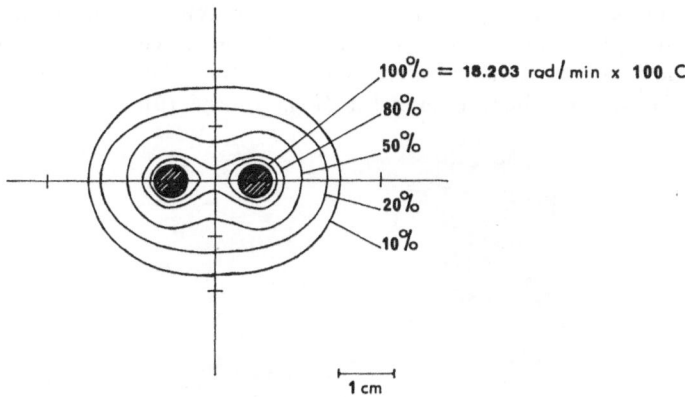

Fig. 11. The same disposition as in Fig. 9. Isodose curves in the plane perpendicular to the two positions and passing for their centers

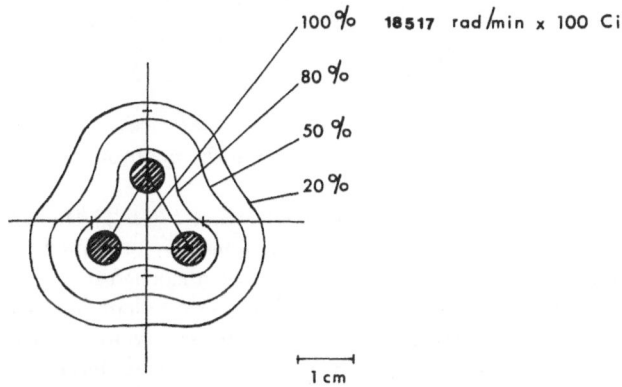

Fig. 12. Source in three parallel positions, at a distance of 15 mm from each other. Isodose curves in the plane perpendicular to the three positions and passing for their centers

in three parallel positions—the isodose curves in the plane at right angle to the sources in their centers.

One observes in these cases a better dose distribution for the treatment of relatively extended tumours.

In order to verify the results obtained, we have produced an analogic dosimetry system.

We have employed not only a lucite phantom, but also a man-equivalent phantom, constituted by a human skeleton inserted in a tissue-equivalent plastic substance, that is in a substance characterized by an absorption of radiation similar to that of brain tissue (Fig. 13).

The phantom's head, as all the body, is subdivided in sheets in which is produced a series of holes; in these holes we have inserted suitable micro-dosimeters, that is micro-condenser ionization chambers and thermoluminescent microrods of LiF (Figs. 14 and 15).

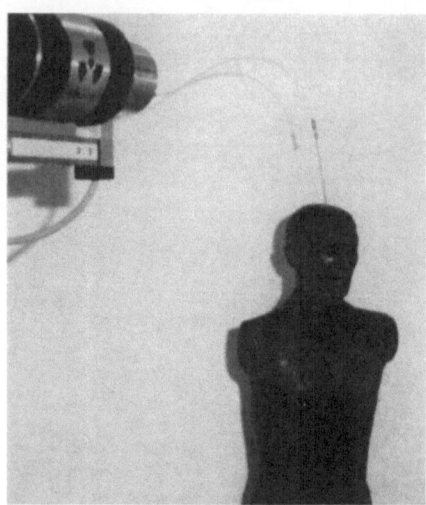

Fig. 13. The source inserted in the phantom's head

Within the limits of experimental errors ($\pm$ 5%) the measurements have confirmed the theoretical determinations previously described.

Moreover, in order to evaluate the dose absorbed from radiosensitives organs, we have employed the same man-equivalent phantom and have simulated the irradiation of a frontal target volume, with the administration of 7000 rads at 1 cm from the source; we have obtained these values:

eye lens	200	rads
pituitary gland	300	rads
thyroid	25	rads
gonads	0.1	rads

It is obvious that these refer only to this porticular situation and may be different for other positions of the source.

However, it is likely that in each treatment doses of this order may be absorbed from the cited organs.

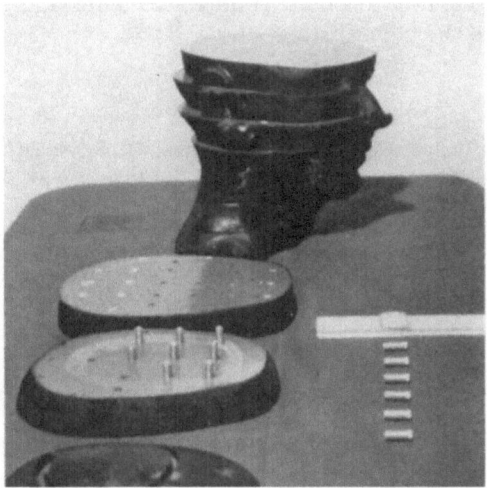

Fig. 14. Sections of the phantom's head with condenser ionisation chambers
inserted

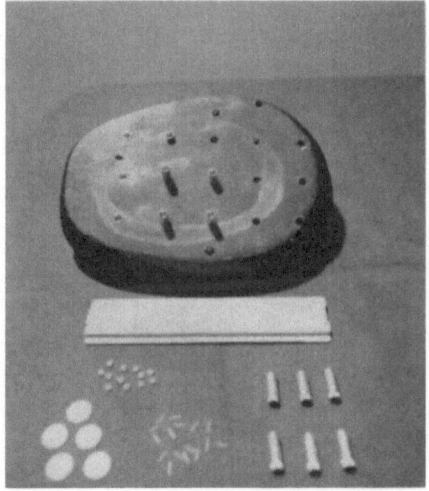

Fig. 15. Section of the phantom's head, with condenser ionisation chambers
and micro-rods and discs of LiF

In our opinion the treatment is justified for patients with brain tumours, for whom the risk of late radioinduced damages can be neglected with respect to the clinical situation.

References

1. Botturi, M., Jucker, C., Tosi, G., Pedrinazzi, G., Scielzo, G. (1970), Impiego di un calcolatore elettronico per lo studio della distribuzione della dose attorno a sorgenti lineari di iridio-192. La Radiologia Medica, LVI, n. 8: 670—684.
2. Mundinger, F. (1958), Beitrag zur Dosimetrie und Applikation Radio-Tantal (Ta[182]) zur Langzeitbestrahlung von Hirngeschwülsten. Fortschr. Röntgenstr. *89*, 86—91.
3. — (1966), Treatment of brain tumours with radioisotopes; in: Krayen-bühl, Maspes and Sweet: Progress of neurological surgery, vol. 1, pp. 101—145. Basel-New York: Karger.
4. — Sauerwein, K. (1966), „Gamma Med" ein neues Gerät zur inter-stitiellen, nur einige Minuten dauernden Bestrahlung von Hirngeschwül-sten mit Radioisotopen, auch intraoperativ anwendbar (mit Film-demonstration). VII. Int. Symp. Neuroradiol., 20. bis 25. September 1964, New York. Acta radiol., Stockholm *5*, 48—52.
5. — (1969), Erfahrungen mit der interstitiellen Brachytherapie mit Ir[192] „Gamma Med" bei infiltrierenden Hirntumoren. Kongreß der Deutschen Röntgengesellschaft, 6. bis 8. Juni 1968, Hamburg. Fortschr. Röntgenstr. *110*, 244—261.
6. — (1970), Brain tumour therapy by interstitial application of radio-active isotopes; in: Paoletti and Yen Wang Monograph: Radionuclei applications in neurosurgery and neurology, pp. 199—265. Spring-field, Ill.: Ch. C Thomas.
7. — Metzel, E. (1970), Interstitial radioisotope therapy of intractable diencephalic tumours by the stereotaxic permanent implantation of Iridium[192], including bioptic control. Confin. Neurol. *32*, 195—202.

Authors' addresses: Prof. Dr. G. B. Delzanno, Centro di Terapia Stereo-tassica „Stella Fossati", Dr. L. Redaelli and Dr. G. Tosi, Servizio di Fisica Sanitaria, Ospedale Maggiore Ca'Granda, Milano, Italy.

Acta Neurochirurgica, Suppl. 21, 265—267 (1974)
© by Springer-Verlag 1974

Regional Clinical Neurophysiology Service, Western General Hospital,
Crewe Road, Edinburgh, Scotland

Towards a Three-Dimensional Brain Model Stored in a Computer

H. R. A. Townsend

With 1 Figure

The project of storing in a computer a three-dimensional brain model is undoubtedly ambitious. The object is to be able to help the neurosurgeon to visualise the structures encounted by a stereotactically directed probe. The technical problems involved in converting between atlas co-ordinates and the actual co-ordinates of a particular stereotactic machine on a particular patient are not very difficult and by themselves seem hardly to justify the use of a general purpose computer, although Dervin, Heywood et al. have demonstrated the possibilities of a dedicated portable mini-computer operating actually within the theatre. Our project must also be distinguished from that of storing in computer memory a brain atlas, in such a way that appropriate sections can be retrieved and displayed with an associated representation of the probe track. A system of this latter kind has been beautifully illustrated by Dr. Bertrand in this symposium.

Techniques for storing line drawings in a computer are fairly well developed and are inherently reasonably economical in terms of usage of computer memory because the information in a line drawing is economically expressed. A crude technique for storing a brain model in a computer is to represent the three-dimensional structures as a series of thick sections, each section being assumed to be homogeneous throughout its thickness and the structures in each section represented as a line drawing. In this way we can store a 25-section model of the first few segments of the spinal cord in about 8,000 words of our computer's memory and from the stored information sections of the cord at any desired angle can be constructed and displayed on the screen of a monitor oscilloscope.

A disadvantage of this method of representation is that in order to discover the points of intersection of the lines in each of the horizontal sections with the desired oblique plane there is no alternative to completely (or almost completely) searching the entire stored representation and this is very time consuming. Where the requirement is simply to display a particular recorded section the job is much easier because

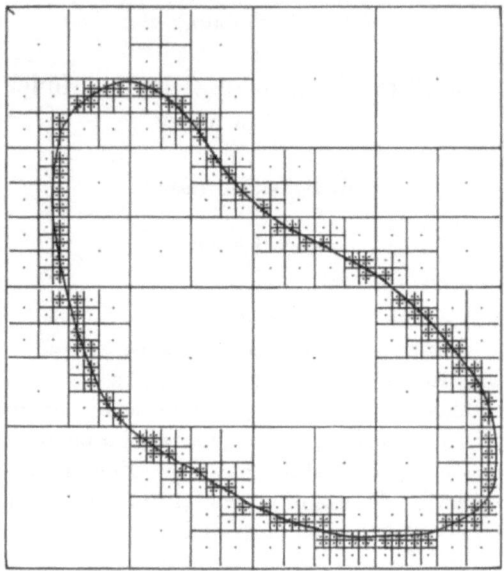

Fig. 1. An arbitrary object is delineated by the technique of successively subdividing an enclosing square

the desired section can be found from an index in one operation, whereas what we are trying to do is to build up a new section from examining a large number of stored sections.

For these reasons we have abandoned this simple internal computer model and started to investigate more sophisticated methods of representing three-dimensional structures. The most promising is the use of a "space occupancy tree". This method of representing objects can most easily be explained by considering the two-dimensional equivalent, although the method itself operates in three-dimensions. The illustration shows a simple figure inscribed in a square. The enclosing square is first divided into four equal squares and the question asked of each subsquare is it (a) wholly outside the figure, (b) wholly inside the figure, or (c) partially inside and partially outside the figure. We now proceed to subdivide those squares which partially contain the object and repeat the procedure on each of the smaller squares so formed. (In the three-dimensional case we start with a cube and subdivide it into 8 sub-cubes, and so on.) With each successive repetition the detail in the region of the edges of the object becomes finer and by continuing to subdivide squares in this way we can define the object as precisely as we wish.

The illustration contains about 600 squares and requires about 900 words of computer memory. A similar three-dimensional model would require about 16,000 words. The representation is accurate to about 1 cmm in a 5 cm cube (125,000 cmm) so the coding is reasonably efficient. A search to determine which of a number of regions contains a particular cmm requires only 6 decisions and hence can be executed very rapidly.

A useful model of the basal ganglia region or of the brain stem and upper cervical region would need perhaps 50,000–100,000 words stored on a magnetic disc. The storage structure can be organized so that the speed of search is adequate to construct an arbitary section in less than a second, and the same technique can be adapted to store details of stimulus responses or evoked potentials.

Summary

A method is described for storing in a rapidly retrievable and reasonably economical form a three-dimensional model representing deep nuclei and physiological responses.

Author's address: Dr. H. R. A. Townsend, Regional Clinical Neurophysiology Service, Western General Hospital, Crewe Road, Edinburgh, Scotland.